LIVING WITH TINNITUS

A clinical psychologist explains how sufferers from 'ringing in the ears' can learn to tolerate the noises in their heads until in many cases they become no more noticeable and distressing than the sounds of breathing.

D0293247

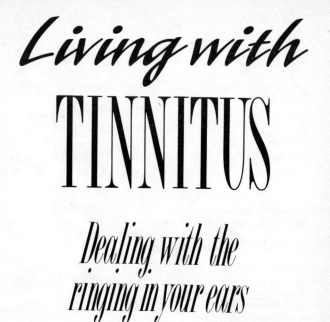

Living with
TINNITUS

Dealing with the ringing in your ears

RICHARD HALLAM

THORSONS PUBLISHING GROUP

First published 1989

© Richard Hallam 1989

Hallam, Richard
Living with tinnitus.
1. Man. Tinnitus. Self-treatment
I. Title
617.8

ISBN 0-7225-1801-3

*Published by Thorsons Publishers Limited,
Wellingborough, Northamptonshire
NN8 2RQ, England*

Typeset by MJL Limited, Hitchin, Hertfordshire
Printed in Great Britain by Biddles Limited, Guildford, Surrey

1 3 5 7 9 10 8 6 4 2

About the author

Richard Hallam was born in London and has spent most of his working life there having graduated in psychology and philosophy from Bangor University in 1965. He subsequently trained in clinical psychology and specialized in behavioural psychotherapy of anxiety-related problems, and was largely responsible for running the first government sponsored nurse-therapy training scheme in behavioural psychotherapy at the Maudsley Hospital in London which led to a national curriculum and new nursing sub-speciality.

He began working at the Royal National Throat, Nose and Ear Hospital in 1981 and has remained there on a part-time basis working in a tinnitus clinic. He has had published over 20 articles on tinnitus, mostly in collaboration with R. Hinchcliffe (Professor of Audiological Medicine) and Simon Jakes (a research colleague). With Simon Jakes he developed group cognitive therapy techniques for tinnitus sufferers and has also run intensive weekend therapy courses.

He is currently teaching clinical psychology at University College London and working as a therapist in the National Health Service and privately.

Acknowledgements

I am grateful to many colleagues and friends who have supported and encouraged us in our work at the Audiology Centre of the Royal National Throat, Nose and Ear Hospital, London. Without Ronald Hinchcliffe's foresight and backing we would not be there at all. Simon Jakes has also played a key role as research collaborator, tinnitus counsellor and friend. Amongst many past and present colleagues, I would especially like to thank Christine Chambers, Dai Stephens, Laurence McKenna and Ross Coles. Bruce Moys and Roy Crabbe gave many helpful comments on the manuscript. Bruce's participation in group counselling sessions is greatly appreciated. My thanks also to colleagues I haven't mentioned who all helped to make this book possible.

Contents

Foreword

Throughout the period of recorded history some men — and women — have been aware of ringings, buzzings and hissings, as well as other noises, in their ears at one time or another. And, characteristically, in these cases there is no sound external to the individual to account for what he hears.

Something like one in four to one in five of us have noticed these noises in the ears at one time or another.

But isn't the body like a machine with noises going on all the time? So what is surprising is not that so many people but that so few people have noticed noises in their ears. Indeed, doctors have shown that, provided we have sufficiently quiet conditions, the majority, perhaps all of us, will be aware of these noises. It appears to be largely a matter of awareness or attention that determines whether or not we notice these noises.

For the most part, even when we are aware of these noises, they do not bother us. Nevertheless, one in every two hundred people are extremely troubled with noises in the ears. Throughout the period of recorded history it is clear that there have been some men and women who have not only been aware of these noises but have complained about them.

Sometimes, but not often, awareness of these noises, or a change in their quality, betokens some underlying disease. It is therefore not unreasonable for people to seek medical advice. More often than not, the doctor will not discover any underlying cause — even after extensive investigations. We are therefore left with a number of individuals who are extremely troubled with these ear noises and for whom there is no medical or surgical treatment.

As is their wont, doctors have given a technical term to these ear noises. They refer to the condition as "tinnitus". There is, however, no special meaning to "tinnitus". All that it means is that the person is experiencing noises in the ears (or the head, for often the sound cannot be localized) for which there is no apparent external source.

Again it is clear from recorded history that a variety of treatments for tinnitus has existed from time immemorial. It is equally clear that the reason for such a variety of treatments has been a failure to recognize why something we all experience has become a source of worry, anxiety, or depression. The awareness relates, as Dr Hallam and his colleagues have shown, to psychological states of attention. Attention to tinnitus is related to stress in people's lives and to the ways in which the noises are interpreted. Indeed, it is on this matter that Dr Hallam and his team have conducted the most enlightening research in recent years. His group has clarified the reasons why tinnitus is a source of complaint. Since this is primarily due to psychological factors, it is logical that psychological methods should be employed to help the tinnitus sufferer.

Dr Hallam sets out to explain tinnitus using words that can be understood by all of us. Not only does he explain tinnitus but he demonstrates that something can be done to reduce its disturbing nature.

Drawing upon his vast research experience and his practical experience in counselling patients, he has been able to produce this book which should be a source of interest and comfort to all those who suffer from tinnitus. It can be strongly recommended not only to tinnitus sufferers but to all those health care workers and scientists who are interested in this topic.

Ronald Hinchcliffe, MD, PhD, FRCP, DLO
Consultant Audiological Physician at the
Royal National Throat, Nose and Ear Hospital
Professor of Audiological Medicine at the
Institute of Laryngology and Otology,
University of London

Introduction

Most of us take for granted that what we hear originates from sounds in the real world. Just occasionally we might notice a whistling or popping in the ears which we know is just a trick of our senses rather like seeing double when pressing on the eye. These illusory noises are a mild form of an experience which can be much more severe and distressing. If the noises are loud and occur frequently they are referred to as tinnitus.

Tinnitus is a medical term for noises in the ears or head which do not originate outside the body. It is a common symptom of ear disorders but it can occur by itself without any other hearing problem. It is a symptom with many causes, and therefore many different medical solutions to the problem must be sought.

No great effort is required to understand what it is like to hear tinnitus noises. The noises are similar to familiar external sounds *except*, of course, that they seem to be located in the head. Therefore, it feels as if there is no way of escaping them. Most of us have been bothered at some time by a buzzing fluorescent light or the noise of machinery. The important difference between tinnitus and these common forms of noise pollution is that there is no one to call in to rectify the problem.

When the problem of tinnitus is described in this way, it seems like a dreadful affliction to most sympathetic observers, so it is surprising that public awareness of the problem is not greater than it is. Surveys of the British population have shown that around 16 per cent of adults hear noises in their ears which last longer than five minutes, and five per cent claim that their sleep is disturbed by tinnitus. For people with poor hearing, noises in the head are often more distressing than the inability to hear well.

There are several plausible explanations for this neglect. First of all, no great medical advances have been made in curing the causes of this symptom, and there are no clear signs that a medical solution will be found soon. Certain drugs eliminate the noises, but they have too many side-effects to enable them to be taken for any length of time. There is no reliable, effective, safe drug for general use, and surgery helps in only an extremely small number of cases.

The mechanism that produces tinnitus is not understood but for the most common type of noise it is assumed to be in the ear itself. The most important parts of the ear are extremely small and encased in bone. Direct examination is impossible, and cutting the nerve to the ear cannot be recommended because it destroys hearing and is, anyway, ineffective. It is not surprising, then, that tinnitus has been a source of frustration to the medical profession, and lack of success does not receive wide publicity.

Second, tinnitus is invisible, and the noises do not literally hurt you. There is no external sign of illness and the affected person appears quite healthy, so does not elicit immediate sympathy. Third, suffering with head noises is more of a psychological than a physical kind of suffering. The noises affect the ability to think, to communicate, and to get by in a reasonable mood.

These difficulties are traditionally in the sphere of the psychologist (or psychiatrist) rather than the doctor. At present, Ear Nose and Throat (E.N.T.) clinics (and general physicians for that matter) do not have ready access to professionals who can assess whether distress is caused by treatable psychological factors. It is not easy for a doctor to say whether the person could be helped by counselling or some form of therapy. If it means making a special referral to a mental health professional (which the patient might in any case resent), the doctor might well think twice about it. In any case, few of these 'experts' are familiar with or take an interest in tinnitus.

It is little wonder, then, that some people who have tinnitus feel abandoned, and it is not surprising that such strong self-help associations have come into existence.

As someone who is a member of one of these mental health professions (clinical psychology) I should explain how I first became involved with tinnitus. The initial moves were made by medical consultants at the Royal National Throat Nose and Ear Hospital in London who felt that little was being done for many of their distressed tinnitus patients. At that time, when the problem was put to me, I confess that the idea of working on the subject was only of mild interest and far from positively exciting. Tinnitus is not the kind of problem that psychologists have traditionally worked on. In fact, some of my colleagues gave me the impression that this was another example of psychology colonizing a new and trivial area of work.

Of course, since then my enthusiasm (shared by my colleagues) has developed and this book is the product of about eight years of research and direct experience of counselling. I am pleased to say that tinnitus has now achieved a much higher profile amongst academics and clinicians.

However, it is still the case that the individual who has passed through medical hands and still suffers with the noises is likely to remain dissatisfied and to have a difficult time getting further help. Tinnitus is rarely related to any life-threatening form of illness and so your doctor may not take it very seriously. He might even tell you that he suffers from it himself!

This book has been written primarily for those who find themselves in this neglected position. Its aims are to present *useful* factual information, to explain a psychological approach to tinnitus annoyance, and to help readers investigate their own tinnitus problem. The book will also assist readers in evaluating the treatments currently on offer.

Be warned that no magic cure for tinnitus will be revealed in the pages to follow. However, I do feel that I have learned something of value from my research and treatment involving hundreds of clinic patients. In the course of this work I have witnessed some dramatic changes in those who felt quite sincerely that tinnitus was eroding the quality of their life. From a state of considerable debility, a person affected by tinnitus can begin to lead a normal life again. I observed also that tinnitus is by no means always unbearable. A few people attending our clinic even *liked* their noises and thought that they would miss them if they went away! Others simply did not give tinnitus a second thought. It had become so much a part of their life that it could be ignored like the sound of their own breathing.

In another and larger group of people I observed a gradual transition from distress to tolerance, and then to acceptance. The process typically takes between three and eighteen months. *I and my colleagues now strongly believe that the normal response to tinnitus is the gradual development of tolerance.* After a period of distress (of greater or lesser degree), it is possible to come to terms with the noises and to live with them as a persisting but relatively minor handicap.

This belief — in the normal development of tolerance — is borne out by the statistics which have been gathered about the number of people who hear noises in the head. The figures show that tinnitus is extremely common. As previously mentioned, approximately 16 per cent of the population are aware of noises lasting longer than five minutes, but not all those affected say that the noises distress them. For example, in only 1-2 per cent of the population does tinnitus definitely disturb a person's way of life. So, even though considerable numbers are affected, the *majority* of people who hear tinnitus noises say that it does not amount to a significant problem.

This does not mean that tinnitus has had no effect at all. Tinnitus is 'real' and the person who experiences noises certainly knows whether they are present or not. However, in the majority of people who hear tinnitus noises, they are tolerable and do not trouble them unduly. This state of acceptance and tolerance may have been hard won following a troubled period. It is this hard won state of tolerance which I, as a psychologist, regard as an acceptable aim for therapy. It is not a cure in the medical sense but it is a cure in the psychological sense.

Why then do so many people with tinnitus reach this state unaided while others feel that the noises are relentlessly hounding them? It is not as easy as it might seem to answer this question but this book will attempt to tackle it. Put most simply, it appears that the noises become a problem when a person pays attention to them. For example, I have encountered several people who had no notion of the 'disorder' until they watched a television programme on the subject! Thereafter, they noticed their own noises which then began to interfere with other activities like reading, relaxing and sleeping. Of course, paying attention is not something that one can easily choose to do or not to do. However, enough is known about the psychological process of attention to help you to develop the ability to ignore the noises.

As one might expect, louder noises attract more attention than quieter ones. However, loudness is by no means the only or the most important cause of tinnitus annoyance (see Chapter 1).

The sensitivity of a person's hearing is also a factor. The person with the most sensitive hearing is *not* the one who is most bothered — quite the reverse. A sensitivity to all surrounding sounds will help to cover up or *mask* the tinnitus. So it is the person with poor hearing who hears their own noises at the expense of the external sounds that matter. For this reason, hearing aids are frequently prescribed to help combat tinnitus (see Chapter 10).

I will expand on these and other psychological aspects of the problem, but this is *not* a medical textbook and, apart from a glossary of medical terms, the physical causes and medical treatments of tinnitus will not be covered. The book should be of most value to those people who have already obtained what help they can from medical sources but still feel that they would like some advice on accepting the problem and coping with it. With this self-help orientation in mind, I provide the reader with some basic factual information which is helpful in understanding tinnitus and its effects.

There are some rating scales and questionnaires to assist in self-analysis, psychological aspects of the process of tolerance are explained, and methods to help you cope with tinnitus are described. Advice is also given on how to deal with tinnitus as an auditory handicap, and masking instruments that are commercially available are discussed in this context.

I hope this book will provide reassurance on several points and set off a chain of events that lead to a lessening of annoyance and distress. Self-help groups have been set up in many countries and they have been very successful in giving much needed emotional support, information and, in some cases, counselling as well (see Chapter 11).

The descriptions I give of psychological techniques should help you to select appropriate professional help if that is what you decide. I trust that readers who get to the end of this book will have gleaned somewhere in their reading the key to a happier relationship with their own 'infernal' noises.

1
For your information

Perhaps the most important and encouraging fact about tinnitus is that in 99 per cent of cases the cause is benign — it is not a sign of serious, life-threatening illness. It does not often get louder over time and, if the severity of the problem is taken to include its psychological effects, then it generally gets 'better' as time goes on.

Is there anything else worth knowing about the noises themselves? Not very much really. Any kind of noise, whatever its quality or loudness, *can* become annoying. Readers who are eager to get on can skip this chapter. However, apart from sheer curiosity about the condition, I believe it is useful to be informed about tinnitus in three ways.

The first is to obtain convincing information about the seriousness of the condition so that fears about becoming deaf, having to give up one's job, or other similar calamities, can be faced squarely and honestly. This is the sort of information that should be provided by your ear specialist.

The second is to obtain information which puts tinnitus 'in proportion'; that is, which gives an idea of how common it is in different age groups, what the typical effects are, whether there are certain kinds of tinnitus that are more troublesome than others, and so on. The third is to find out what can be done to help a person to cope with tinnitus, the different kinds of help on offer, and how they are supposed to help.

This chapter is about the second reason for being informed about tinnitus — factual information to put tinnitus in proportion. In subsequent chapters I suggest ways of assessing your noises and collecting useful information about them. This is a preparation for the chapters giving a deeper understanding of tinnitus annoyance. Information about professional help and self-help follow on later.

How many are affected?

'Normal tinnitus'

The body is not a completely silent place and so a certain degree of 'tinnitus' is normal. Sounds result from the mechanical movement of muscles, bones, blood and air. Moreover, our ears, like any mechanism, are unlikely to be perfect and perform without any background hum at all. These background bodily noises become noticeable in especially quiet surroundings. If a person (with normal hearing) is placed in an extremely quiet environment (for example, a chamber which is insulated against outside sounds), it is highly likely that a hiss, buzz, whistle or some other 'sound' will be heard. It is supposed that in everyday conditions, these background noises are masked by the louder sounds of the environment — they are simply not heard. In exceptionally quiet surroundings, as in the sound-insulated chamber, 'we hear the silence'.

Another common and *normal* experience is a noise in the ears which follows exposure to a very loud sound such as hammering or disco music. This usually lasts a few minutes. Something like half the population readily acknowledge that they have 'had' tinnitus at one time or another.

'Significant tinnitus'

'Normal tinnitus' can become 'significant' if attention is drawn to it. In other words, some sufferers (we don't know how many) may simply be unduly concerned about something that everyone else takes for granted. However, the most likely reason for tinnitus to become significant is its getting louder or more frequent. Louder noises are more noticeable and, therefore, may become bothersome.

How common are these louder and more persistent forms of tinnitus? Several surveys have been carried out to obtain this information. It has been possible to reach a figure which excludes all the minor forms of tinnitus caused by loud sounds, catarrh, water getting in the ears, and so on. Tinnitus which *lasts longer than five minutes* affects about one in six persons. Are *continuous* noises more troublesome than less frequent noises? Yes, this is generally true as can be seen from the results of a survey of British householders in 1981 (see figure 1). The duration of noise counted in this survey varied from 'continuously present' to 'less than one minute, less than once a week'. Almost no-one was bothered in the latter group. The most affected people were those who had continuous noises or frequent bouts of noise lasting an hour or more. However, *only about a third of these most affected people were bothered by noise to a significant extent.*

Looking at it another way, the majority of adults with continuous noises were bothered only 'slightly' or 'not at all'. So, the amount of time the noises are present is important, but this is not the whole story because there are many people with continuous noises who are not unduly bothered.

There are several ways of explaining this awkward fact away. People who are bothered may have *louder* noises or they may be more vulnerable to noise — for example, if they are living alone

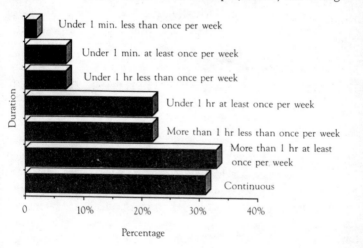

For each group, the bars show what proportion of people are bothered 'a great deal' or 'quite a lot'. The duration varies between 'continuous tinnitus' down to 'less than a minute, less than once a week'.

Figure 1
Number of people disturbed by tinnitus according to its duration and frequency.

or feeling low. Another possibility is that some people who hear continuous noises are no longer bothered because they have learned how to ignore them.

The effects of tinnitus according to age and sex

If we just consider tinnitus lasting longer than five minutes then the older you are the more likely you are to experience it. The proportion of adults affected rises from 7 per cent (21-30 year-olds) to 17 per cent (61-70 year-old group). For 'continuous noises' the watershed is the age of 40. Below this age it occurs in about 1 per cent of the population but it shoots up to 8 per cent in the over sixties. We have to conclude that, for many of us, tinnitus is part of the experience of growing old.

The number of people for whom tinnitus has a *severe effect on the quality of life* is of course less than this. The size of this severely affected group increases with age as well, but older and younger *women* seem to be more bothered than their male counterparts.

The effect of tinnitus on the ability to sleep normally is *not* related to age — it occurs with the same frequency at all ages. But once more, for some reason, older and younger women are more likely than men to have their sleep affected by tinnitus.

Loudness and other qualities of the noises

It is natural to expect that if the noises are especially loud and persistent they will attract a lot more of our attention. A quiet tinnitus may be tolerated for years but then cause trouble if it suddenly starts to get louder. But we have found that this whole question of loudness is more complex than it appears at first sight. We know that loud *external* sounds are not always unbearable so we have to ask what is different about *internal* sounds. A pneumatic drill operator will tolerate levels of noise that make normal speech impossible. Some factory workers tolerate a very noisy environment for hours without obvious discomfort. The loudness of these external sounds is far greater than the loudness of any internal sounds as far as we can estimate them. A second point is that loudness is a relative quality. In the dead of night in the countryside, an owl's hoot can sound very loud indeed;

amongst city traffic it would not be noticed. This is one reason why tinnitus seems so much louder in the middle of the night and prevents a return to sleep.

The loudness of tinnitus varies a great deal between individuals and so this is an obvious quality to assess in order to see whether the level of distress reflects the measured loudness. Assessments of loudness are commonly made in a tinnitus clinic. Loudness can vary from hour to hour or day to day and so more than one assessment may be needed. Tinnitus pitch is usually assessed at the same time. The pitch refers to whether the tinnitus sounds like a high note (e.g. a squeak, whistle, tinkle) or a low note (e.g. drone, rumble, hum). Some tinnitus is a mixture of sounds of different pitches in which case it may sound like a roar or a hiss.

Assessment by matching in a tinnitus clinic

The chief method of measuring the pitch and loudness of tinnitus is to compare it with an external sound produced by a sound-generator. The patient sits in a very quiet testing room and headphones are placed over the ears. Sounds are then played into one ear — usually the one with the better hearing. In *loudness matching* the patient has to adjust the volume of the sound until it exactly equals the loudness of the tinnitus noises. In another test, the sound is increased until it just drowns out the tinnitus noise. This is called the *minimal masking level* of the sound.

In pitch matching the patient has to say whether the tone that is played into the ear is of a higher or lower pitch than their own noise. The technician then adjusts the sound, higher or lower, until the pitch match is just right. This test can only be done when tinnitus does *have* a pitch and even then the test is not easy to perform.

The pitch and loudness matches are not of great value in medical diagnosis. For example, it is not possible to diagnose the cause of an ear disorder on this basis. However, the loudness match and minimal masking level may be of help in deciding whether a masker is likely to be of benefit (see Chapter 10). If a tinnitus can be masked only with a very high volume of sound (or not at all) a masker would be of little value. The masking noise would be unpleasantly loud and possibly even damage the hearing mechanism.

Assessing loudness with rating scales

The following method is based on my own research into tinnitus loudness. The object is to find an external comparison sound that is *just louder* than (or about the same loudness as) the tinnitus noise. So if you have tinnitus, compare each of the following sounds to your own tinnitus beginning with the softest. When you reach a sound that is at the right level look at the number of the sound. This is your score for loudness and you can see below how many other people with tinnitus have a quieter or louder noise than yourself. If the loudness of your tinnitus varies, you might like to select two numbers to represent the softest and the loudest values. The figures should be regarded only as a general guide.

The following sound is the SAME LOUDNESS or JUST LOUDER THAN my tinnitus:

The sound of my own breathing	Score 1
A quiet watch near my ear	Score 2
The motor of a fridge in the room I am in	Score 3
The sound of a normal conversation	Score 4
Hailstones on a window I am sitting beside	Score 5
Vacuum cleaner I am using	Score 6

Refer to Figure 2 to find out how many people with tinnitus have a quieter or louder tinnitus than yourself.

The average score for hospital patients attending our tinnitus clinic was between 3 and 4; that is, below the level of normal conversation. In another, larger, survey of almost 1,000 tinnitus sufferers, the loudness of the noises was rated on a scale similar to ours. It was also found that the average rating of loudness was just below the level of normal conversation. Of course, there was quite a range, with 14 per cent saying it was no louder than a whisper and 8 per cent comparing it to the sound of a low-flying jet. These judgements of loudness, even though they are subjective, agree reasonably well with loudness measured in a more objective way by comparison with actual sounds delivered to the ears (the method of loudness matching described above).

Your tinnitus is:

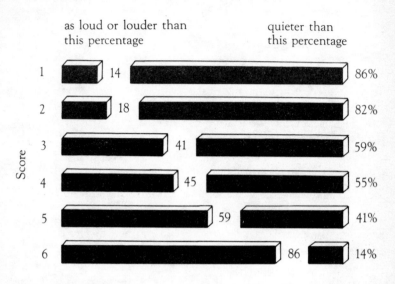

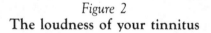

Having decided on your loudness score (opposite), this chart tells you what proportion of people with tinnitus have a noise that is as loud *or* quieter *than your own noise.*

Figure 2
The loudness of your tinnitus

Quality of tinnitus and its effects

Do different kinds of noise produce different degrees or types of suffering? Is it easier to ignore some types of noise than others? Are certain noises more likely to produce insomnia? I have to admit that there is little to tell the reader in answer to these questions. A considerable amount of research has come up with remarkably little in the way of positive results.

In one study carried out at a world-famous tinnitus clinic, 1,800 people rated the severity of their tinnitus on a scale from one to ten (ten equalled an 'extremely severe tinnitus'). Over half the group rated between 7 and 10 — that is 'very severe'. The researchers were surprised to find that these ratings of the severity of the noises were not related to how loud they were (according to the loudness match assessments). Nor could any relationship be found between the severity of the **noises and** whether the tinnitus was constant or fluctuated in **loudness** or whether it was high or low pitch.

Of course, tinnitus may be 'severe' for quite different reasons. Some people say that the noises are distracting and affect their concentration, others that the noises make them feel emotionally distressed, and others complain only that their sleep is disturbed. These different causes of severity should really be considered separately when investigating their relationship to the quality of the noises. The lesson from the research mentioned above is that when you compare the loudness of one individual's tinnitus with that of another's this doesn't seem to explain why one person is more distressed than another, or rates their tinnitus as 'more severe'.

So although loudness may seem to be the crucial factor on a day-to-day basis, this fact has not yet been scientifically demonstrated with proper loudness-match tests. You may believe that you suffer with your noises *because* they are loud. People who are not affected often think that they are less bothered because their noises must be *quieter* than average. These beliefs may be unfounded. Now obviously enough, loudness must be of *some* importance because if tinnitus was so quiet that it could be masked virtually all the time by daily sounds, it wouldn't be a problem at all.

However, I believe that tinnitus sometimes appears loud because a person is annoyed and distressed - not that they are annoyed and distressed because it is loud. I have also come to the conclusion that a loud tinnitus does not *have to be* annoying. Once the brain has stopped 'taking note' of tinnitus (see Chapter 5) the noises can be ignored even though they are loud. So, in the early stages of living with this problem, variations in the daily loudness might make quite a difference to how you feel. But at a later stage, when the noises are better accepted, loudness variations may become less important or even without significance.

Because the loudness of the noise often seems to be its most important quality, we have devised a diary for monitoring tinnitus loudness on a daily basis. This can be found in Chapter 4. Daily monitoring is a useful way of checking whether an assumption about tinnitus is correct. For example, it is possible to check whether the level of annoyance really does coincide with loudness levels by looking at this carefully and systematically.

Summary

By any standard, tinnitus is a problem of considerable social proportions and a significant cause of personal suffering. It is more common in the middle-aged and elderly who may well have a double handicap if they also have poor hearing. Poorer hearing means that the masking effect of environmental sounds is diminished and so the effect of head noises is accentuated. Tinnitus can also add to the effects of poor hearing because it can intrude when a person is trying to pay attention to what others are saying.

A lot of figures have been presented in this chapter and their significance is not yet fully understood. However, there are some main points. Tinnitus is common but the majority of people who experience it do not consider it to be a major problem. As one might expect, if the noises are very infrequent they are unlikely to be bothersome.

Tinnitus becomes more common after the age of 40. By middle age, there is probably a cumulative effect of wear and tear on the ears due to ageing, exposure to loud noises, the side-effects of certain commonly used drugs, viral infections, and other causes. The severity of a tinnitus cannot be easily understood in terms of loudness, pitch, or other quality of the noise. The loudness varies a great deal between individuals. The average is somewhat quieter than the level of a normal conversation.

Nearly all the causes of tinnitus are of a benign nature, and tinnitus can be regarded as a natural hazard of modern life and of the process of ageing.

2
How tinnitus can affect you

What people with tinnitus have in common is a noise in the ears or head. Beyond this, they are likely to share some typical psychological effects of the noises. If, however, we analyse the problem in more detail, we find great variation in the way tinnitus can affect a person. In this chapter I can do no more than give a general description of typical problems. A lengthy interview would be required to go further than this and make a proper analysis of a person's difficulties. This is something I do routinely in the tinnitus clinic in which I work. Nevertheless, by means of the questionnaire and diary explained in the following chapters, you will be able to make a start on your own self-analysis.

There are several reasons for taking care over the analysis of your tinnitus difficulties. First of all, to find the best way to cope with them, you need to know exactly what you are facing up to. The importance of this will become apparent when you read Chapter 8 on cognitive techniques. Secondly, it is useful to estimate how far along the road to adaptation and tolerance you have travelled.

Recognizing the fact that you have already learned to ignore the noises even a little should encourage you because it is a sign that further progress can be made. The full development of tolerance may take several years and may occur so slowly that you hardly notice that you are overcoming the problem.

Lastly, it is important to separate out the effects of tinnitus from other problems. If you have been experiencing psychological problems for some time, the onset of tinnitus may have brought this to light. It is not easy to stand at a sufficient distance from yourself to be able to weigh up the relative importance of tinnitus and other problems. For this reason, I do not attempt to guide you in this respect. If you believe that problems unrelated to tinnitus are important in your case, it is advisable to seek expert opinion. Even if your reaction to tinnitus is *not* complicated by additional problems, it should be obvious that as a person with a certain style of dealing with stress and with various life experiences of illness, deafness, and related matters behind you, your response to tinnitus will be an individual one.

Your psychological response to tinnitus is likely to fall into one of three main patterns (1) emotional distress, (2) intrusion of the noises into your thoughts and daily activities, and (3) insomnia. Most likely you will have a mixture of all three with the emphasis on one or the other. Insomnia is the most variable response affecting about 50 per cent of sufferers.

Emotional distress

The authors of a recent survey of tinnitus club members concluded that the most important task for the tinnitus counsellor was to deal with the emotional effects of the noises. Certainly, it is emotional distress that is likely to lead to a call for help. Your emotional reaction is in part secondary to the ways tinnitus interferes with your work and leisure. But often the emotional reaction is primary and related to what tinnitus *means* to you. If you see tinnitus as calamitous you will experience fear and anxiety. If you see no end to tinnitus you will feel depressed. If you resent your employers (or doctors or life in general) for bringing this on your head, you will feel resentful and angry. The range of emotional reactions that tinnitus can provoke is large. I discuss this topic further in Chapters 6 and 8.

The chain of events that leads to your emotional reaction can be complex. Take just one example from my own professional experience to illustrate this. A man gradually became depressed after developing tinnitus. This event coincided with the death of his young god-daughter. His retirement was due shortly and he was worried by the fact that his depression would not lift and would ruin not only his own retirement but, more important to him, his wife's enjoyment of their old age together. Seeing things in this way added to the stress of these events, and tinnitus appeared to be the main culprit. However, it is clear that to entirely blame tinnitus for this state of affairs would neither be accurate nor helpful. It is because a person's life is often troubled in different ways that help is needed to sort out the many causes of distress, and to address each one separately.

The trap this man fell into was to see tinnitus as the source of all his difficulties. A common and understandable error of this type is to believe that any difficulty with concentration or memory is due to the way the noises intrude into your thinking. Tinnitus *may* do this, but an anxious or depressed mood can also have these effects. As your emotional distress lessens, so your ability to think clearly without distraction should improve as well.

The effect on your family or social relationships is again variable. Your behaviour may have changed, or have a tendency to change for brief periods, with no outward sign of the cause. How do family members know that your increased irritability or unsociability is the result of tinnitus? For that matter, how do you know for sure yourself that this is the true reason for the way you feel? How much explaining is worthwhile, knowing that your family has heard it all before? You may feel both *guilty* for not being so lively and light-hearted as before, and *resentful* that your family does not seem to be as sympathetic as perhaps they might be. All this is a recipe for a mixed-up emotional state which needs careful thinking about to find the best solution.

Tinnitus is capable of producing the most extreme state of despair. Amongst a group of tinnitus club members 7 per cent had contemplated suicide. In my own questionnaire survey of 100 hospital outpatients, 8 per cent responded that life would not be worth living if the tinnitus persisted; a further 19 per cent said that this statement was partly true for them. If a deep depression sets in it may seem impossible to get back to normal. But the prognosis for recovery from depression is good, especially if it is a secondary reaction to your noises. Do not let the sense of hopelessness hold you back from seeking help.

Intrusiveness of the noises

A difficulty in understanding speech is one of the most common problems associated with tinnitus. You are likely to experience this in situations which would for anyone demand more concentration than usual, such as having a conversation in a noisy social gathering. Your ability to localize speech, that is, knowing what direction it is coming from, may be impaired as well. Voices, too, may sound distorted.

These difficulties are made worse by the additional presence of a hearing loss. It is not yet known how much of the blame lies with tinnitus or with hearing loss. Both must contribute to listening difficulties. Listening, as opposed to hearing, is a mental activity and, like all mental activities, it is less efficient when your attention is distracted by irrelevant noises. It is this capacity of tinnitus to distract attention which probably results in a loss of the powers of concentration. Your ability to think while reading or doing other mental tasks may be interrupted by attention to the noises. One student I knew was unaware of his noises while reading until he came to a difficult passage. This question of attention is discussed in more depth in Chapters 5 and 6.

Many pastimes require good hearing as well as concentrated listening. These include watching television, listening to the radio, and the appreciation of recorded music. These activities can therefore be spoilt by tinnitus. However, as time goes by, the distracting effects can lessen. I encountered one musician who was able to ignore his noise (a constant tone) while playing his instrument. When I asked him for the pitch of the tone he listened for a moment and replied B flat. It appeared he had not bothered to make a note of this before, surely a sign that he was paying little attention to it.

In some occupations, like teaching, tinnitus is more of a handicap than in others. But I am reluctant to generalize too much. For some sufferers, intense mental concentration can provide relief.

The intrusiveness of the noises depends to some extent on the volume of background sounds. In one survey, it was found that the worst times were early morning, late evening or night-time. Less than 2 per cent said that mid-morning was the worst time, probably because this was a time of absorbing activity and greater ambient sound. It was also found that women who worked were less troubled during the day than women who didn't work, showing the importance of these influences.

Insomnia

Insomnia can take the form of difficulty in getting to sleep, of waking in the night, of early morning wakening, or of all three. It is puzzling that insomnia is sometimes the main or only problem, while for other individuals sleep is unaffected. In fact very little is known about insomnia caused by tinnitus. It is likely that there

are differnt types of tinnitus insomnia — for example — sleeples-
ness brought about by worrying thoughts, waking induced by loud
tinnitus, and early morning wakening associated with a depressed
mood.

About a quarter of all persons who report tinnitus claim that
tinnitus wakes them up at night. One survey showed that the
louder the noises the more likely it was that there would be a
difficulty getting to sleep or being woken up.

Broken sleep can develop into a habit which is difficult to break.
Getting up in the night may be followed by a ritualistic visit to
the toilet and the making of a hot drink, habits which may eventually keep the insomnia going. It is obviously extremely trying
to be woken up in the dead of night when the noises sound louder
anyway and you do not have the opportunity to distract yourself
by physical activity. In Chapter 9 I describe some psychological
techniques for developing a normal sleep pattern. These are alternatives to the use of sleeping tablets — which may be helpful in
the short term but tend to lose their potency after several months
of continued use. Patients attending tinnitus clinics often mention worry about dependence on sleeping tablets (or about their
side-effects) as a reason for seeking help.

Stages of tolerance

If you follow the typical sequence of reactions to tinnitus, you
can be assured that tolerance of the noises will develop in time.
I try to explain what I mean by 'tolerance' below. Some people
develop tolerance quickly and others do so slowly. The reasons
for this are being investigated by researchers and I can report some
preliminary findings. Of interest to many is the question whether
their noises will get louder over time. If this were to happen you
might feel that you could never develop tolerance for them.

A survey was conducted recently on a random sample of
voters from the British electoral register. The members of the
sample who reported tinnitus were asked about the history of
their noises, that is, whether there had been changes in their
loudness or in the annoyance they had caused. It seems that
when the noises *start suddenly* the loudness remains unchanged
in around 70 per cent of the cases. The loudness gradually
decreases (or the noises end) in about 20 per cent and there is

an increase in loudness for 10 per cent.

When the noises have a *gradual onset* (i.e. they don't begin suddenly but slowly develop from an almost imperceptible level) there is a somewhat greater chance of the noises continuing to get louder. This happened for 20 per cent of the cases. As before, in 70 per cent, the loudness remained unchanged and in 10 per cent there was a decrease or an end to them.

In a different survey, persons affected by tinnitus were asked to look back over the previous 10 years and say how the loudness of the noises had changed. On average, there was a slight increase but it amounted to only half a division on a 10 point scale. This probably means that for the majority there was no change at all.

To sum up, if your tinnitus follows a typical course, the chances are good that the loudness of the noises will not change. If the loudness increases that doesn't necessarily mean that you will automatically get more distressed. As I have explained elsewhere, you cannot simply equate loudness and annoyance. More people are distressed by the *fear* of tinnitus getting louder than are ever distressed by a loud tinnitus.

The survey of voters quoted above did look at trends in annoyance as well. Overall, there is strong evidence of annoyance decreasing over time. Of those who were *severely annoyed* at the beginning (a minority of the total) 70 per cent showed a lessening of their annoyance. This is encouraging but it still leaves some severely affected individuals showing no improvement.

I have found that the development of tolerance typically takes between about three and eighteen months. I am not sure how far the process of ignoring the noises can ultimately be taken. I can certainly point to some individuals for whom the noises hardly seem to exist in any psychological sense, though if the noises were to be measured by matching and masking techniques they would be indistinguishable from the noises heard by tinnitus sufferers.

The emotional effects diminish first, followed later by improvement in concentration. Difficulty in listening and understanding the spoken word may persist indefinitely if hearing loss is also present. It is important to emphasize that improvement in the way tinnitus affects you can take place even though there is no actual change in the noises. This is borne out by measurements taken before and after psychological therapy for tinnitus. Distress lessens, but the pitch and loudness matches of the noises (see Chapter 1) stay the same.

I have drawn up a sequence of stages in the development of tolerance, as follows. You will not necessarily follow this precisely.

STAGE ONE

- Persistent awareness of the noises except during sleep and masking by louder sounds.
- Frequent worrying and depressing thoughts about tinnitus.
- Concentration on mental tasks difficult to sustain for more than a few minutes.
- Absorbing activities provide only slight distraction.
- Insomnia severe (if present). Cumulative sleep loss in some cases necessitating medication.

STAGE TWO

- Intermittent awareness developing - especially during absorbing activities. There are moments when you are aware that you have *not* been aware.
- Improvement in concentration reflected in increasing engagement in habitual activities.
- Beginnings of emotional acceptance; the implications of the noises no longer seem catastrophic.
- Gradual return to normal sleep pattern (if disturbed).

STAGE THREE

- Awareness mainly limited to periods of tiredness, stress or quietness.
- Noises intrude mainly when listening and mental concentration are important (at social gatherings, the theatre, lectures, etc.)
- Noises annoying rather than emotionally distressing.

STAGE FOUR

- Attention rarely given to the noises. Attention limited to periods when they are louder than normal or you are reminded of them.
- Noises do not intrude into normal activities.
- Emotional acceptance achieved — the noises are neither pleasant nor unpleasant.

As an exercise, it is worth noting down all the ways in which you were affected by tinnitus when it first started and what thoughts you had about it at that time. If you wish, rate each effect on a scale of severity from one to ten. Now consider the present situation and re-rate yourself. You are likely to discover that your tolerance has increased. Further change in a positive direction can be expected.

3
The Tinnitus Questionnaire

The following questionnaire was developed over a number of years for use in a tinnitus clinic based at a hospital. We interviewed several hundred patients attending the clinic. Some were distressed by their noises; others had learned to tolerate them or had never been troubled. Through our experience of asking these patients how they were affected and what tinnitus meant to them, we devised a questionnaire which covered the themes that cropped up most frequently. The questionnaire is now given out in advance of the interview so that the checked items can be discussed in more depth.

The questionnaire has gone through several versions. Instructions for filling it in and scoring it are provided below. It yields a useful summary profile of your reaction to tinnitus and helps you to pinpoint the main difficulties. The answers to certain questions assess your beliefs about your noises and these can give a lead in applying cognitive therapy techniques (see Chapter 8).

The answers to the questions contribute to several different scales (A, B, C, D, E, F). The range of low, medium and high scores for each scale is given below together with an explanation of what each scale means.

Instructions

The purpose of this questionnaire is to find out whether the noises in your ears or head have had any effect on your moods, habits or attitudes. Please answer each question by indicating whether the statement is True, Partly True, or Not True for you. Just circle the appropriate answer. There are no right or wrong answers. Just answer the way you feel. Please answer all the questions.

SCORING: Next to the answers there are several columns, A, B, C, D, E, and F and for each answer there is a number, 1, 2, or 3. Put the number that goes with your answer on the dotted line (---) in the columns. Usually there is just one dotted line but occasionally there are two. If so put the number in both places. When you have completed the questionnaire add up your score separately for each column. You will end up with six scores, A to F. The meaning of the scores is explained below.

#	Statement	True	Partly true	Not true	A	B	C	D	E	F
1	I can sometimes ignore the noises even when they are there	1	2	3	.	.	.	.	.	---
2	I wake up more in the night because of the noises	3	2	1	.	---	.	.	.	.
3	Your attitude to the noises makes no difference to how it affects you	3	2	1	.	.	.	---	.	.
4	Most of the time the noises are fairly quiet	1	2	3	.	.	.	---	.	.
5	Because of the noises I have difficulty in telling where sounds are coming from	3	2	1	.	.	.	.	---	.
6	The way the noises sound is really unpleasant	3	2	1	.	.	.	---	.	.
7	I feel I can never get away from the noises	3	2	1	.	.	---	.	.	.
8	Because of the noises I wake up earlier in the morning	3	2	1	.	---	.	.	.	.

		True	Partly true	Not true	A	B	C	D	E	F
9	I worry whether I will be able to put up with this problem for ever	3	2	1	.	.	.	----	.	.
10	Because of the noises it is more difficult to listen to several people at once	3	2	1	.	.	.	.	----	.
11	If the noises continue my life will not be worth living	3	2	1	----	.	.	.	.	.
12	Because of the noises other people's voices sound distorted to me	3	2	1	.	.	.	.	----	.
13	I wish someone understood what this problem is like	3	2	1	.	.	.	----	.	.
14	I worry that the noises will give me a nervous breakdown	3	3	1	.	.	.	----	.	.
15	Sleep is my main problem	3	2	1	.	----	.	.	.	.
16	I find it harder to use the telephone because of the noises	3	3	1	.	.	.	.	----	.
17	I am able to forget about the noises when I am doing something interesting	1	2	3	.	.	.	.	----	
18	It takes me longer to sleep because of the noises	3	2	1	.	----	.	.	.	.

					A	B	C	D	E	F
19	The noises are loud most of the time	True 3	Partly true 2	Not true 1	.	.		---		.
20	Because of the noises I worry that there is something seriously wrong with my body	True 3	Partly true 2	Not true 1	.	.		---		.
21	The noises distract me whatever I am doing	True 3	Partly true 2	Not true 1	.	.	---	---		.
22	The noises have affected my concentration	True 3	Partly true 2	Not true 1	.	.	.		.	---
23	Because of the noises I am unable to enjoy the radio or television	True 3	Partly true 2	Not true 1	.	.	.		---	.
24	It will be dreadful if these noises never go away	True 3	Partly true 2	Not true 1	---	.	.	---		.
25	I have more difficulty following a conversation because of the noises	True 3	Partly true 2	Not true 1	.	.	.		---	.
26	I find it harder to relax because of the noises	True 3	Partly true 2	Not true 1	.	---	.	.	.	.
27	A stronger person might be better at accepting this problem	True 1	Partly true 2	Not true 3	.	.	---	.	.	.
28	I am more liable to feel low because of the noises	True 3	Partly true 2.	Not true 1	.	.	.	---	.

						A	B	C	D	E	F
29	I sometimes get very angry when I think about having the noises	True 3	Partly true 2	Not true 1		.	.	.	---	.	.
30	I am more irritable with my family and friends because of the noises	True 3	Partly true 2	Not true 1		.	.	.	---	.	.
31	I often think about whether the noises will ever go away	True 3	Partly true 2	Not true 1		.	.	.	---	.	.
32	I can imagine coping with the noises	True 1	Partly true 2	Not true 3		---	.	.	.	.	.
33	My noises are often so bad I cannot ignore them	True 3	Partly true 2	Not true 1		.	---	.	.	.	.

SCORING KEY

A high score means greater disturbance by tinnitus

Scale	A	B	C	D	E	F
HIGH SCORE	8-9	16-18	9	36-42	15-18	8-9
MEDIUM SCORE	5-7	11-15	6-8	23-35	10-14	5-7
LOW SCORE	1-4	6-10	3-5	14-22	6-9	3-4

Scale A. This scale is in some ways the most revealing. A high score indicates helplessness about ever learning to cope with the noises. This belief inevitably leads to pessimism about the future. One of the purposes of this book is to show you how these feel-

THE TINNITUS QUESTIONNAIRE

ings can be combatted, and to convince you that it *is* possible to learn to live with noises despite their continued presence.

Scale B. This scale indicates the extent to which tinnitus has affected your capacity for 'rest and relaxation'. If a high score is obtained, then the section of the book concerning relaxation train-ing and insomnia will be especially relevant (Chapter 9).

Scale C. A high score here indicates that it is hard for you to accept that *anything* will make any difference to the way tinnitus affects you. You might have acquired this attitude for a variety of rea-sons. For example, if you see tinnitus as a purely medical problem then psychological attitudes make no difference. A medical cure is the only acceptable solution. On the other hand, you might have discovered that *nothing does* make a difference one way or the other. This is rather unlikely. If there is something that makes tinnitus *worse*, there is probably something that makes tinnitus *better*, and this may be partly under control. If you also obtain a high score on scale D then your attitude probably does make a difference to how it affects you.

Scale D. This scale measures the more common emotional effects of tinnitus and the beliefs that tend to go with them. This is why this scale has the most items. It is on this scale that we would expect most change with the passage of time. Many of the beliefs included here are those that you may hold when tinnitus first starts and you are feeling at your lowest point. These beliefs will be examined more deeply in the chapters on acceptance and seek-ing help. During cognitive therapy (Chapter 8) the validity of the beliefs is directly questioned.

Scale E. You are likely to obtain at least a medium scare here, espe-cially if you also have a hearing loss. Tinnitus diminishes your ability to hear speech and other sounds distinctly. These effects are most resistant to psychological approaches to tinnitus. However, this is not to say that nothing can be achieved in this area.

Scale F. Some people have the ability to 'put the noises to one side' and ignore them while they are doing something interest-ing. A low score means you have come a long way in this direc-tion. High scorers should not feel too discouraged because this ability can be acquired.

4
Self-analysis II: the tinnitus diary

The tinnitus diary will help you to discover what makes tinnitus more or less 'severe' on a day-to-day basis. For you, to be 'severe' might simply mean to be 'loud'. In fact, with a little careful observation, you should be able to distinguish the loudness of the noises from how noticeable, annoying or distressing they are. Even if the loudness of your noises seems constant, the *effects* of tinnitus will certainly vary in some way from day to day.

About one quarter of people with tinnitus report large fluctuations in loudness. Whether or not the loudness changes in your case, you will notice tinnitus more at certain times than at others. Tinnitus is often more noticeable when you are tired, stressed, or feeling emotionally upset. Your bodily position (lying, sitting, or standing) can make a difference too. As I have mentioned before, tinnitus is less noticeable when you are absorbed by an interesting activity or simply in a happy mood.

These variations in tinnitus and its effects can be monitored by keeping a diary. If the information is recorded in the manner described below, the diary becomes a way of testing out ideas about what it is that makes the tinnitus better or worse. A diary can also be useful over a longer period for monitoring the effect of a change of diet or a new medicine. Having identified something that *does* affect the tinnitus, its influence can sometimes be lessened by a change in your lifestyle or habits. It is possible, of course, that the changes recorded in the diary will look completely random, and they may well be so if these changes are related to some obscure aspect of your body chemistry. Even so, a diary can be useful to prove that something is *not* making your tinnitus worse. Disproving a strongly held but unjustifiable belief has the effect that changes in tinnitus become less meaningful and therefore easier to tolerate (see Chapter 6).

Ratings of loudness should be made separately from ratings of annoyance. Loudness and annoyance may be related but they are not identical. On many occasions, I have seen a person's annoyance reduce while the loudness of tinnitus remained the same.

I have always recommended using the following seven point scales for diary recording. Seven degrees of tinnitus severity is usually about as much as anyone can distinguish.

For loudness:
1 = extremely quiet (you can barely hear it)
7 = as loud as your tinnitus has ever been

The points in between 1 and 7 represent degrees of loudness. So, for example, 5 might mean a moderately loud noise. The exact definition of each point of the scale is not so important as the fact that you stick to the same definitions from day to day, otherwise the numbers won't make any sense at all.

For annoyance:
1 = not at all annoying
7 = as annoying as your tinnitus has ever been

The same sort of considerations apply here as mentioned above. Make sure the numbers make sense to you.

I suggest that the diary is completed not more than three or four times a day. The times chosen for recording should be decided in advance. Either pick definite times, for example 8.00 a.m., 12.00 noon, and 8.00 p.m., or make an overall judgement for the morning, afternoon, and evening. If your tinnitus varies a lot, you could simply rate the worst levels for each period. There are no rules about this except to stay with the same method once you have started. Ideally, you should make your ratings in a notebook you have drawn up for this purpose and jot the figures down at the time that you are judging the tinnitus. If you leave it for a day or more, your memory is sure to play you false.

Keeping a diary might have the undesirable effect of increasing your awareness of the noises. This might happen if you are assessing the noises very frequently. For this reason, I suggest that a diary is kept for an experimental period and for a particular purpose only. If you introduce any change into your diet, medicines or lifestyle, then the diary should be kept for a few weeks before the change and kept going for at least a few weeks after the change has been made. To make doubly sure of any effect of the change in habit you can go back to the original conditions, for example, to eat the supposedly offending foodstuff, and record again for a few weeks.

The completed diary might look something like this:

DAY	Monday	Tuesday	etc
Early morning (*loudness*)	4	5	
Early morning (*annoyance*)	7	6	
Daytime (*loudness*)	3	5	
Daytime (*annoyance*)	2	2	
Late evening (*loudness*)	5	5	
Late evening (*annoyance*)	5	5	

In addition to the ratings of loudness and annoyance it will be useful ro record certain other items of information. Sleep disturbance can be noted by a suitable code, for example, getting to sleep-GS; waking in the night-WN; or early morning waking— EW. Events that stress you can also be recorded, such as work stress-WS; but it is important to remember that these events should be recorded *at all times* and not just when the tinnitus is bad. Unless this is done it will not be possible to discover whether at certain times work stress is *not* followed by worsening tinnitus. In fact, a heavy workload might even be a blessing at times by taking your mind off the noise.

What can be done with all this information? To make sense of it the figures should be added up or put on to a graph. For example, the ratings could be added up separately for morning, daytime and evening to find out the best and worse times of day. Then, if a change is introduced, such as taking a new drug, the same figures can be added up for the weeks following the change. Another way of looking at the results is to add up the daily totals for loudness and annoyance and put them on a graph as follows:

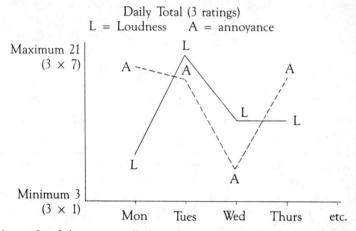

Daily Total (3 ratings)
L = Loudness   A = annoyance

A graph of this type will show up a general trend in the ratings over time; cyclical effects may become apparent. For example, it might become obvious that weekends are a good (or bad) time and it might be worth reflecting on the reasons for this.

Now suppose a connection is sought between, say, drinking coffee, and the loudness or annoyance of tinnitus. Here is one method for working this out. First, decide what ratings count as tinnitus being 'good' or 'less severe' (say 1-4) and then what counts as tinnitus 'bad' or 'more severe' (say 5-7). You will have to add up the following figures:

Mornings coffee is drunk:

........Number of times tinnitus good   = _____ (a)
........Number of times tinnitus bad   = _____ (b)

$$\text{Percentage of the time tinnitus bad when coffee is drunk} = \frac{(b)}{(a + b)} \times 100$$

Now this should be compared for mornings when coffee is *not* drunk:

........Number of times tinnitus good   = _____ (c)
........Number of times tinnitus bad   = _____ (d)

$$\text{Percentage of the time tinnitus bad when coffee is not drunk} = \frac{(d)}{(c + d)} \times 100$$

All this might look a little complicated but it is just a question of working out percentages. Finally, you have to compare the percentages. If the difference between the mornings that coffee is drunk and not drunk is rather small (say tinnitus severe 50% of the time versus 60%) you might not think it worthwhile making this change to your lifestyle. How you make these judgements is up to you of course.

Another exercise that may prove interesting is to look at the relationship between loudness and annoyance. Just as for the coffee example you compare the percentage of the time that tinnitus is annoying (e.g. rating 5 or over) when the tinnitus is soft (rating 1-4) or loud (rating 5 or over).

You can go on to look at the effects of work stress or any other event that has been coded. It may become obvious that a certain event is associated with greater annoyance. This might suggest to you changes in lifestyle that could minimize the severe periods. If there is no sense or pattern in the figures then this is the moment to put the diary away and give up on this tack.

Food, drugs and other substances that may be related to tinnitus loudness/ annoyance

This subject is included here because you might wish to use the diary to investigate the effects of foods or medications. You might think that a drug you are taking is responsible for making your tinnitus worse. Alternatively, you might have reason to believe that your diet is lacking essential ingredients and the diary can be used to test the effects of positive changes in your nutritional intake.

If you believe that prescribed drugs are producing or intensifying your noises do *not* stop taking them without seeking your doctor's advice. It may be necessary for you to take them even if they do have adverse effects on your noises.

I will labour the point again that there are many different causes of tinnitus. In a certain proportion of sufferers, probably not more than 5-10 per cent, sensitivity to the toxic effects of foods or drugs, or allergies, contribute to the cause of tinnitus. For a very small number of affected individuals these factors might make all the difference between hearing the noises and not hearing them.

Medicinal drugs

The number of medicinal drugs that have tinnitus as a *possible* side-effect is very large indeed. Some drugs can potentially produce hearing loss as well as tinnitus. Only a very small fraction of patients who are prescribed these drugs that could damage the ear ('ototoxic drugs') suffer these unfortunate side-effects, and the drugs are not normally prescribed at levels that produce damage. When side-effects do occur there may be several reasons for this. Sensitivity to drugs varies a great deal, so what is safe for you may not be safe for someone else. There may have been some pre-existing (and undetected) malfunction in the ear before the drug was prescribed which could increase vulnerability to drugs, and drugs taken singly without harm may become toxic in combination with other drugs. It has even been shown in research with animals that drugs that are harmless to the ear in a quiet environment can damage it in a noisy one.

I will not give you a list of drugs that have been known to produce tinnitus as a side-effect. This could be unnecessarily alarming. The list includes some antibiotic, diuretic, analgesic, and psychotropic drugs. By far the most commonly used drug known to produce tinnitus is aspirin. In the past, some doctors judged the maximum dose of aspirin by increasing it until the patient heard noises. Small doses are unlikely to produce any permanent change in tinnitus. If you take aspirin regularly for headaches or other minor complaints, it may be worth substituting a non-salycilate drug.

Quinine, used in the treatment of malaria, is also known to produce tinnitus.

Several types of antibiotic can produce tinnitus in susceptible individuals. One young woman attending our clinic developed tinnitus in this way. She was bitterly resentful of the doctor who had prescribed it but in fact her case was exceptional, and her life had been saved by prolonged antibiotic treatment. An unavoidable degree of risk attaches to all drug treatments.

Non-medicinal drugs

It is widely claimed that such universally ingested substances as caffeine (in tea, coffee and cola drinks), nicotine (in tobacco) and alcohol can intensify tinnitus noises. If you enjoy these substances or if you are dependent on them, giving them up will be a major decision. First you will want to know whether they influence your tinnitus in the short-term. This can be discovered without too much hardship by rating your tinnitus on, say, alternate half-day or full-day periods when you do or do not indulge yourself.

To be more convinced of an effect you will have to give up your habit altogether for a month or more. This won't be easy especially if you are a heavy smoker. Giving up might make you feel tense and irritable, a frame of mind in which your tinnitus might seem more annoying anyway. To make a fair comparison with your tinnitus before giving up, it is perhaps best to wait until your mood returns to normal before restarting your diary. A recording of two to three weeks should then be sufficient to assess any improvements.

Diet and allergy

The role of diet in health is a controversial subject. Only a small number of tinnitus experts place a great deal of emphasis on diet or food-related sensitivities or allergies. It is possible that a lack of essential minerals, vitamins or other nutrients is responsible for an inefficient or tinnitus-producing ear, but diet interacts with other influences on your general health and so the topic is a complex one. Further reading is suggested at the end of this book.

An allergy is a hypersensitivity of your immune system to certain substances. Your immune system is responsible for defending your body against disease, especially invasion by viruses or bacteria. In some people, apparently harmless substances such as grains of pollen or food proteins can trigger the immune system into action. The symptoms of allergy may include skin rashes, swollen red-rimmed eyes, coughing and wheezing, 'hay fever', gastric discomfort and many others. Ear symptoms, including tinnitus, are commonly mentioned in the literature on allergy. If you suspect allergy then seek expert advice. The existence of food allergy is usually established by experimenting with diet as other methods of diagnosis are unreliable. You will need to keep a tinnitus diary if you decide to test out the effects of making changes in your diet.

Stress and environmental factors

If there is a pattern in your diary annoyance ratings according to the time of day or day in the week, this might give you a clue to the reasons behind your fluctuations in annoyance. The following influences could be important when tinnitus is either especially annoying or not bothering you at all:

- Bored or busy? How absorbed are you by other activities at these times
- Effects of environmental sound? Are you bothered mainly in quietness? Do loud sounds in your environment have a masking effect or do they increase the loudness of your noise?
- Harrassed or stressed? Are you overloaded — by work, managing boisterous children, or straining to listen to something? How much of this is unavoidable or is due to the way you interpret the situation? Are you expecting to be bothered by tinnitus and are you having depressing thoughts about it when the noises are 'severe'?
- Is tinnitus preventing you from enjoying a favourite activity such as listening to music or just relaxing?

The diary should enable you to uncover the main reasons for being more distressed at one time than another. It is important to note when the noises are *not* bothering you just as much as when they *are*. Jotting down a few notes about your activities and thoughts at the time of making the diary ratings can assist you in your self-analysis. The value of this exercise will become apparent when you read later chapters.

5
Accepting tinnitus: the importance of attention

What does it mean to 'accept' tinnitus and what is the point of it? A sceptic might say 'tinnitus is *always* there — I *have* to accept it.' I will try in this chapter to explain what I mean by acceptance, and demonstrate that this attitude makes common sense as well as theoretical sense. The idea of 'acceptance' may be hard for you to grasp if you have not already gone through several stages with your tinnitus. I have heard a client remark that he really understood 'acceptance' only after he had already achieved it. At an earlier stage he thought he had accepted tinnitus but later realized that he hadn't really done so. You can't consciously 'decide' to accept tinnitus and then expect matters to improve immediately. But I believe that it's possible to put some effort into this process of acceptance in a roundabout way.

The first step is to acknowledge that tinnitus is present, that it probably won't go away, and that it can be a handicap in certain situations. To accept tinnitus is then to regard it as completely unworthy of further thought.

But you may find yourself thinking about tinnitus constantly. Why do I have it? What has caused it? Is the cause serious? Will it go away? Will it drive me crazy? These questions, and a great many others besides, are all perfectly reasonable. What is not reasonable is to continue to ask yourself the same questions day after day. It is then that the noises are brought into the forefront of your attention giving you a sense of their unrelenting persistence. It is as if a permanent in-tray of questions never gets emptied, and so tinnitus remains in awareness, reminding you of this fact.

Before going on to consider the kinds of unfinished business that keep tinnitus in awareness in this way, I will explain a little more about the psychological process called 'attention'. What I have to say implies that tinnitus is an attentional problem as much as it is a medical problem.

The process of attention

What I am trying to explain here is a basic fact of our psychological survival. Try to imagine everything that you are capable of sensing — through hearing, seeing, touching, smelling and feeling. You *never* experience all that you are capable of sensing at one and the same time. This would be overwhelming. Typically, you notice one thing after another — a door banging, an itch, the sun suddenly appearing, and so forth. To attend means to bring something into your conscious mind (your 'attention system'). You attend, first, to those things that occur in a mildly surprising way (for example, the door banging) and, second, to those things that are useful to you in the activity you are pursuing. So in writing, I pay attention to the words flowing from the movement of my pen and to the thoughts I might be having.

You are normally only consciously aware of one thing at a time. When my attention is distracted by a door banging I might continue to write 'automatically'. For that fraction of a second when the door bangs I am not paying attention to the words in my field of vision. There are many activities that we do automatically without paying full attention, including driving a car. For several seconds at least, a driver's thoughts may be far away from the road.

Just as there are two reasons for paying attention, there are two reasons why you *stop* paying attention to events. First there are the boring, repetitive or meaningless events that are happening all the time. A ticking clock, the sound of your own breathing, traffic noise, or a refrigerator hum, are all sounds of this kind. Most of the time, too, you are unaware of your bodily position or bodily sensations. These sensory events are opposite in nature to the new and interesting happenings that catch your attention.

The second kind of inattention consists of ignoring the events that you need to help you carry out activities automatically. In driving a car automatically, you still need to use your eyes, even though you don't pay full attention to the road. You are able to use visual information without actively paying attention to it. It is a remarkable ability to be able to ignore the information coming into your senses while at the same time monitoring what's going on and using information as necessary. You could not survive without this ability because you need to be flexible in switching your attention from one thing to another. So for example, while day dreaming on the motorway, it is important to notice the signs of an accident or potential accident ahead. The flashing police sign is picked up on 'automatic' but then you focus your full attention on driving.

We can think of tinnitus as a disorder of attention. In terms of our psychological survival, a tinnitus noise should belong to the category of boring, repetitive events which have no meaning. It is not an event which should continue to surprise you and grab your attention. Neither is it useful as sensory information to control automatic habits. And indeed, what I have observed, working in a tinnitus clinic, is that in the majority of cases, tinnitus does eventually recede into the background of the conscious mind, only coming into the forefront of attention when it is perhaps louder than usual, during stress or tiredness, or in quietness. This state of relative inattention to the noises contrasts with the state of affairs when tinnitus is first noticed. As a new experience, it is constantly in conscious awareness, intruding into activities like reading a newspaper or relaxing on the sofa. It is as if tinnitus is constantly announcing 'I'm still here' when a person knows full well the tinnitus is still there. This is experienced as a feeling of tinnitus 'persisting'.

Notice that some continuous sounds, like the sound of your own breathing are perfectly acceptable and always in the background. Listen to it now and you will realize that there is sound associated with your breathing. You only become aware of this on rare occasions. Many different factors are involved in alerting your attention and I will discuss these later. The point I wish to make here is that there are stages in the process of learning to ignore tinnitus. Stages, in other words, in the level of attention you give to tinnitus.

Attention and tinnitus

What I am proposing is that a tinnitus noise can be regarded as similar to an external sound. It is something to which you may or may not attend. When you first notice tinnitus it might seem like an everpresent intrusion from which there is not a moment's peace. Sleep may be impossible for nights on end, and so literally there is not a moment when tinnitus is not heard. However, even at this stage, it cannot be true that your waking life is totally taken up with tinnitus. It is necessary to pay attention to other events simply to talk, to make decisions, avoid traffic, and so on. You are never a complete robot, automatically controlled and unaware of what you are doing except for listening to the noises.

In these early stages, some people deliberately keep themselves busy with activities that take up their conscious attention (thereby excluding tinnitus, however momentarily). The activities that are chosen for this purpose often include home decorating, housework, taking the dog for long walks, gardening, or mending the car. The more your attention is taken up by these activities, the less your mind is occupied with tinnitus.

Later on, the stage of so-called 'complete awarenss' gives way to periods of inattention. Suddenly, you notice that you have *not* noticed tinnitus for a period of time. Later on still, tinnitus is noticed only at certain times, as mentioned above, during stress,

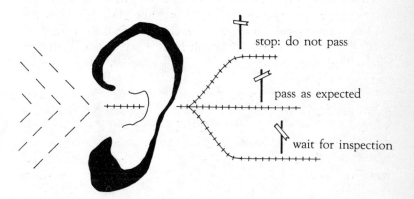

stop: do not pass

pass as expected

wait for inspection

This diagram illustrates how sounds are analysed and how the information is dealt with. (1) Familiar, *meaningless* sounds are *stopped* and the information is not passed on to enter your awareness of influence your behaviour. (2) Familiar, *meaningful* sounds are passed on to control your behaviour without the need for your constant awareness.
(3) Intense, unfamiliar or puzzling sounds are inspected with full awareness.

Figure 3
Analysis of sounds according to their significance.

tiredness, or in quiet surroundings. I believe that the process of ignoring the noises can be taken even further than this. I have come across some people with tinnitus who could block the noises out of their conscious mind in the same way that they could ignore the sound of their own breathing.

One way to picture levels of attention to external sounds is to visualize them being carried along three railway tracks, as in Figure 3. At the end of the first track all information is stopped; it is not passed on to the conscious mind for further analysis. The second track, with its raised signal, allows the information to pass by — everything is going according to plan. The information is understood and used and there is no need to pay attention. If necessary the signal can be lowered and the information examined. The third track has the signal lowered. The information is investigated. What is it? What does it mean? Where shall I send it? This represents the most intense level of attention comparable to the state when you first became aware of the tinnitus noises.

This tracking and routing of external sounds (and other sensory information) is conducted by the brain as part of its normal operation. You cannot decide *not* to pay attention any more than you can decide that in the next five seconds you are *not* going to think about pink elephants (try it). The gradual decrease in levels of attention to irrelevant information is an automatic process and you must trust in the power of your brain to perform it. The way that you, through your conscious thinking mind, can influence it has to be indirect as you will see later.

My hypothesis is that the same processes of attention are involved in learning to ignore tinnitus noises even though they are internally generated unlike external sounds. How long does this progressive decrease in levels of attention take? I cannot give a definite answer to this question. Amongst other factors, the length of time probably depends on your threshold of hearing, the actual loudness and quality of your noises and your mood at the time. I find that it's not unusual for the progression to an acceptable degree of inattention to take eighteen months.

What happens to the loudness of the noises over this time? From the research that has been carried out so far, I have no reason to believe that there is any change at all in the noises as far as we can measure them by matching techniques. However, it is possible that as the noises recede into the background, they will appear to be subjectively a little quieter.

How long it takes to 'get used' to head noises and accept them is extremely variable. For some people who develop tinnitus, it is not something to get unduly troubled about. They will perhaps go to see a doctor once or twice before thinking no more about it. For others, and these make up a proportion of attenders at a tinnitus clinic, there may be little sign of a lessening of attention over several years.

In the next chapter I will talk about the various factors that influence the level of attention to tinnitus. In this way I hope to explain why it is that some people come to terms with the problem quickly while others remain distressed for many years.

6
To attend or not to attend

Why is it that one person can ignore head noises while another seems always to be aware of them? If the ideas I put forward in the last chapter have some truth in them, then we can look for an answer in the *usual* reasons that people pay attention or don't pay attention to everyday sounds. There are two main reasons for paying attention, as I have already said. First, there may be something about the quality or timing of the sound which is new or unexpected. Second, we pay attention to sounds because of what they mean to us. In some cases, it is because the meaning is puzzling that we pay attention. Let's look at how these two reasons could be relevant to the amount of attention you give to your noises.

Sensory qualities of the noises

Loudness. The quality overriding almost all others in our everyday world is the volume (loudness) of sound — or so it seems. Even loud sounds must be surprising to get our attention. The short sharp shock of a car backfiring is especially effective. However engrossed we are in what we are doing we are likely to stop briefly and swivel our head in the direction of the sound. But equally loud sounds that are more or less continuous do not attract our attention in the same way. Because they are continuous they are no longer surprising. Loud familiar sounds can be tolerated quite well. Large numbers of people spend 35-40 hours a week working in noisy environments. Work is possible because the worker does not *listen* to the noises and, therefore, the mind is free to engage on the job that has to be done. Active listening is what makes noises annoying and fatiguing.

Tinnitus noises vary a great deal in loudness from one person to another. The loudness can also vary from moment to moment. Following on from the arguments above, it should be easier to ignore a noise of constant loudness than one which fluctautes. However, other things being equal, the louder the noise on aver-age, the longer it should take to learn to ignore it.

Some people who have a constant noise wish for just a few moments complete silence or, as they see it, for a moment's peace. I am not at all convinced that this would supply the needed respite. I predict that a few moments silence now and again would make it harder rather than easier to tolerate the noises. Indeed, surveys have shown that people with frequent intermittent noises are just as likely to get annoyed as people with constant noise.

A period of distress and annoyance is sometimes triggered off by a change in the sensory qualities of your noises. What was once familiar, now becomes new or 'surprising' again and so the process by which your brain ignores the noise sensation has to start all over again, and this takes time. When it is the loudness that increases, your noises will not be so easily masked by ambient sound and so the amount of time that you are aware will increase also.

Instead of an increase in loudness, a new noise might appear or the old noise might change in pitch. Any change will require a new spell of adaptation. It is not uncommon to find a person who is adapted to one noise but not another. It is often the more unpredictable noise that is more annoying. A change that is espe-cially feared by some is a new noise developing in an unaffected ear which is then thought to signify a worsening condition. In this case, the difficulty in ignoring the noise has more to do with its meaning than its surprisingness.

Pitch and other qualities. There is very little evidence to suggest that the pitch or other qualities of tinnitus help to explain why one person is more annoyed than another. Low pitch rumbles and high pitch whistles can be equally difficult to tolerate. It seems to be an individual matter. The word you use to describe your noise might highlight some obnoxious quality but there is no guarantee that what you perceive as 'screeching' or 'grinding' will sound the same to another person.

The meaning of tinnitus

It might seem too obvious to state that you pay attention to those events that are meaningful to you. But sometimes you have only a general notion that something is important without quite knowing what it means or whether you will be able to deal with it. You are likely to pay close attention to these puzzling events in an attempt to make sense of them. Once you are able to fit a puzzling event into a familiar framework you are usually able to accept and ignore it. A squeaking noise at night can be forgotten once you know that it is a door swinging on its hinges and not a burglar entering the house. To accept tinnitus, therefore, means making sense of it in a particular way so that you are satisfied that all the important questions you have about it have been settled. It will then become much easier to ignore.

Tinnitus as a puzzle

When you first notice tinnitus, you may think it is caused by the plumbing, a faulty electrical appliance, or the rumble of lorries in the distance. Sooner or later it dawns on you that the noises are in your head because they follow you around. A visit to the doctor may establish that the noise is tinnitus. If this term is unknown to you, you will want to find out more about it and perhaps make enquiries of friends and relatives. At the end of what is often a lengthy process of information gathering, the noise is pigeon-holed and, if you feel there is nothing worth doing about it, gradually accepted.

Tinnitus remains puzzling if it is surrounded by continued uncertainty. Some people believe that there *must* be a discoverable cause and that the cause can be remedied. It seems unfair. 'How is it that *I*, at my age, having eaten health foods all my life and avoided tobacco and alcohol, have developed this problem?' It is distressing for some patients to hear that their doctor is unable to suggest a definite cause or offer a definite treatment. If this degree of uncertainty is unacceptable, some patients will spend much time and effort seeking second, third and fourth opinions. They will always be on the alert for new cures.

I don't wish to give the impression that a second opinion is never worth seeking. But having seen two or maybe three reputable ear specialists and received a similar opinion, a limit must be drawn. Otherwise, tinnitus will remain in the centre-stage of attention. Unfortunately, there are always some unscrupulous 'experts' who promise the hope of a miracle solution where none exists. This attitude of living in hope, if encouraged too much, adds significance to the noises making them more difficult to ignore.

Part of the puzzle of tinnitus may reside in events surrounding it in the past or in uncertainty about its possible future consequences. In either case there is unfinished business to be dealt with and so the tinnitus cannot be put away and ignored. Let us consider the past and future aspects separately.

Meaningful past events

You may feel that the 'cause' of your tinnitus can be pinned on human rather than natural causes. If negligence or error were involved, it is natural to blame someone and feel angry about this. Your employers may have been irresponsible in failing to provide ear protectors or for failing to cut down on excessive noise levels when it was within their power to do so. Individual doctors are sometimes blamed for prescribing certain drugs or for carrying out procedures on the ear carelessly or in error. Ear syringing is commonly suspected as the 'cause' of tinnitus though establishing this with certainty is very difficult.

Accepting tinnitus in these cases would amount to giving up on this, often justified, anger. When it is justified, compensation may be sought through legal channels. It is important to have resentment acknowledged even if things are not taken this far. All reasonable means of redressing wrongs done should be pursued. Beyond this, the rehearsal of justifications for outrage serves only to perpetuate and add to the distress that tinnitus causes. Tinnitus is a constant reminder of these unresolved feelings and so the noises remain permanently in the focus of your attention.

If you are pursuing a claim of compensation for damage done to your ears, the likelihood of being able to ignore the noises will be much reduced. Unfortunately, the legal process can take many years to complete. Meanwhile, tinnitus is a reminder of wrongs done and therefore cannot be seen to be less than it is. Tinnitus has to be troublesome to justify the claim — and tinnitus obliges. I am not making a strong case here against starting legal proceedings — which in any case are mostly pursued on account of hearing loss and not tinnitus — but I feel I ought to record my own limited observations on the matter so that you can weigh up the pros and cons.

Tinnitus is associated with past events in other ways too. The memory of being extremely distressed, perhaps more distressed than ever before, is associated with the noises. That the noises could reduce you to such a low point can be a blow to your self-esteem. You are not 'the same person' and it might come as a shock to learn that something as outwardly trivial as noise could do that to you. Therefore, accepting the noises and tolerating them might require a slow process of coming to terms with this new self-image.

Meaningful future events

Tinnitus may come to signify an uncertain and unpleasant future. The most common worries are about physical and mental health. You might, for example, worry that you are developing a brain tumour or that you will gradually become more and more deaf. You may fear that tinnitus will get louder, that new noises will appear, or that tinnitus heard in one ear will spread to the other. If you allow these worries to mount up, it is feared everything will get too much and you will have a nervous breakdown. This, ultimately, leads on to financial worries, and you imagine normal working becoming impossible.

I cannot claim that these worries are entirely unfounded. However, I remind my clients that everyone is faced with a small probability of future unpleasantness of some kind. Normally, we do not worry about these events until they arrive — for one thing we cannot predict them, except in a general way. As I pointed out earlier, the probability that your noises will get louder is not high — usually they stay about the same. Also, I repeat again, you cannot make a simple equation between loudness and annoyance.

There is of course a possibility that the disorder affecting your ear will get progressively worse. Your doctor should know which those disorders are and to what degree this might happen to you. After examining you and performing various diagnostic tests, your doctor will be able to offer expert and usually reassuring advice about the future implications that may be worrying you. If exposure to environmental noise has been a factor, this can be avoided in future by the use of ear plugs or ear defenders when sound levels are high. Tinnitus is a chronic ailment but not one that carries a high risk of deteriorating health. The distress it produces lessens over time and so the general picture is one of improvement. However, distress is undoubtedly prolonged by *worry* about future ill-health.

If you have reached the point of having fearful thoughts of going out of control, ending up in psychiatric care, with your family destitute, it would not be surprising if tinnitus became impossible to ignore. The anxiety engendered by these thoughts has a real effect on the physiology of your body and so the fear of losing control seems to be confirmed by numerous symptoms. A vicious cycle sets in. This may be fed by the effects of sleeplessness which, if severe, leads to exhaustion and a failure to cope adequately with daily affairs.

It is often the previously healthy and contented person who has most difficulty in coming to terms with the emotional effects of tinnitus. Age, too, is important. An elderly person might feel that some ill-health is normal, and just be grateful that it is not something more serious. The young are more affronted by tinnitus (unless, of course, they have heard noises as long as they can remember and accept them as normal).

A stage of emotional distress should be expected with tinnitus but I have seen so many people pass through it that I am confident in telling new sufferers that they *will* gradually feel better. It is the *meaning* of tinnitus that I am talking about — its past, present and future implications which are crucial in maintaining attention to the noises. This is why cognitive techniques described in Chapter 8 have been employed to examine and dispute these meanings of tinnitus in the interests of diminishing their significance for you.

Personal factors and paying attention

So far I have talked about general reasons why attention to the noises is maintained. In addition we have to consider whether it is something about you, your circumstances, mood, or personal problems that is the critical factor. I have found that some people who are distressed by tinnitus undoubtedly do benefit from counselling which explores problems that go beyond tinnitus itself. It is generally suspected that your pre-existing mood plays a large part. If tinnitus develops when you are already in a low mood or under stress, then the noises will be harder to ignore.

Tinnitus is even described in some psychiatric textbooks as a symptom of anxiety — probably because being anxious and being annoyed by noises often go together. In my opinion, anxiety and other moods do not cause tinnitus. The association between the two comes about, I believe, because an anxious or depressed person is more likely to have thoughts of a worrying or depressing nature about tinnitus and is generally more distractable.

Some of my clients admit that they have always been worriers. They are not surprised that they worry about tinnitus but that realization doesn't make it any easier to *stop* worrying about it. In fact, if they stopped worrying about it, no doubt some other problem would come to the fore.

I have found that counselling clients about problems that seem quite unrelated to tinnitus is often the first essential step. One effect of dealing with other problems is to increase a person's general resilience. Thereafter, in a more hopeful frame of mind, tolerance of the noises develops as well. The onset of tinnitus sometimes forces you to reassess the way that you have dealt with your life generally. Grumbling problems that have been put aside are dealt with. If they are successfully resolved your mental well-being can increase despite the presence of tinnitus.

There is the exceptional person who finds solace in having a medical disorder, especially one that cannot be cured. Tinnitus is not too convenient for this purpose because, being invisible, it is unlikely to elicit much sympathy. However, I suspect that tinnitus does occasionally serve this purpose and that the complaint has its own rewards. Although this is often hard advice to take, I suggest to clients that they think carefully about the way their tinnitus also affects family members. I suggest that rather than letting others know how they feel, they find other ways of coping when they are distressed. Sympathetic attention is a confirmation of illness. The important step to take is to think of yourself as 'well' and to act on that assumption.

Tinnitus is unacceptable!

It is all very well, you might say, to be told that the noises are untreatable and I must accept them — but I can't continue as I am — I can't work, I can't relax, and I can't sleep. In any case, I know that a cause cannot be found for my tinnitus and I accept that but I can't stop worrying about it!

There is indeed a stage at which you might feel desperate for help. The only help that seems worthwhile is to get rid of the noises. All I can say at this point is that (1) you are probably mistaken if you think that all your distress can be laid at the door of tinnitus; (2) tinnitus might be uncontrollable, but your reaction to it and perhaps other sources of distress *are* controllable; (3) your fears and worries may be unfounded and can be overcome with counselling and support; (4) others have faced the same difficulties as yourself and surmounted them — why not you?; (5) the great majority of people who have head noises come to terms with their condition.

In some cases, the handicaps associated with tinnitus are a threat to pursuing your occupation. For example, it may be difficult for you to sit in committee meetings or attend social gatherings where several people are talking at the same time. Tinnitus is more of a handicap when good hearing is especially important for your occupation, for example, for singers, musicians, sound engineers, and teachers.

I do not wish to underestimate these problems but the implications may not be quite as serious as first thought. An audiological assessment is needed to sort out how much of the problem is due to a hearing loss and how much is due to tinnitus. With some ingenuity, ways may be found of limiting the effects on your work. The main point is that your ability to ignore the noises is likely to increase with time. You are unlikely to be able to see how far you can develop that ability while you are still distressed. Getting rid of the noises or leaving your job may not be the *only* solution worth considering.

7
Seeking help

Your first step in seeking help will almost certainly take you to your general practitioner and from there to an ear specialist. You will be counselled along the way or, at the very least, receive advice and information. It is unfortunate that almost everywhere in the medical world the expert dealing with your medical symptom is separated physically and by theoretical training from the expert who might help you with your psychological reaction to it.

The reception you get from your doctor when you stray from your medical symptoms and begin to talk about what you *feel* about them obviously depends on a number of factors. Some doctors, by reason of their personality or training, will be helpful. There are other doctors who have little knowledge of tinnitus and the time they give to the consultation may be brief. Consequently, your reaction will be pleasure, relief, or disappointment, as the case may be. One or two individuals I have met felt completely rejected. It is at this early stage when the noises are a new experience and their implications are uncertain that you are most receptive to information — and also most vulnerable. Let us now consider the doctor's role and attempt also to put ourselves in the doctor's shoes.

The doctor's role

You will probably want to know from your doctor or ear specialist the likely cause of tinnitus, whether the cause can be treated, whether the noises can be suppressed, and whether in a general sense, you can be helped to feel better. Your doctor will help you by taking your noises seriously, and you should begin to feel that at least someone understands the problem. A thorough medical examination should allay your anxiety about possible causes of tinnitus. Through matter-of-fact questioning, audiological testing, and tinnitus matching, your doctor should reinforce your knowledge that tinnitus is *real*. This form of reassurance is especially important if you mistakenly believe that the noises are a symptom of mental disorder. It is possible that you hear your noises as tunes or melodies. This is not in itself that unusual, and is by no means a sign of madness.

The doctor is in a position to provide information about the loudness of the tinnitus, the degree of hearing loss, if present, and the relief (or increased disturbance) produced by environmental and masking sounds. Your doctor should correct you on any grossly mistaken fears about the noises if he or she spends sufficient time to uncover them. One well-renowned otolaryngologist suggests asking the following question — while watching the patient's expression! 'How would you feel if I discovered you did have a very serious disease!' This might seem a little underhand but many patients are reluctant to admit fears to a doctor in case they sound absurd. Many think that by expressing concern about a serious illness, they are offering a diagnosis in competition with the doctor. Other patients limit their communication to strictly objective information for fear of being regarded as 'neurotic'. A good doctor should be able to pick up on these cues and respond sensitively to your, perhaps unspoken, concerns. A doctor should note, for example, that a patient who is evasive when offered a diagnosis or who does not seem reassured by good news may well be harbouring the belief that there is something seriously wrong.

You are also likely to have specific questions concerning the prognosis — will the tinnitus ever go away and what can be done to prevent a deterioration of the disorder or symptom? The doctor's task, and it is not an easy one, is neither to alarm you unnecessarily by concentrating on the symptoms too much nor to treat you like a moron who is unable to understand anything about the nature and treatment of tinnitus. You will not want to feel that important medical facts are being concealed. Facing the most likely outcome that tinnitus will not go away leads to less anguish in the long run than being left in suspense about this important question. Fortunately, in the majority of cases, tinnitus noises do not get louder over time and so this bit of reassurance can be given.

Doctors cannot state with certainty the outcome of any disorder but they should be able to give you an informed best estimate of the probabilities. However, given their Hippocratic oath, it comes as an admission of defeat to say that they have no medical treatment to offer. Very often you will be sent for more tests or offered a different drug simply because your doctor dislikes sending you away in a distressed state. But, as we shall see later, the alternative to being told that there is no appropriate medical treatment for tinnitus is not simply that you will 'just have to live with it'. The point is that it is not *just* tinnitus that you are living with. This is where counselling comes in.

To clarify what I am saying, there are two components to any illness. First, there is a malfunctioning or damaged system together with the bodily sensations that result. Tinnitus is a prime example of an experience produced by a disordered system. Pain, likewise, is the result of certain kinds of malfunction or damage. The *second* component of illness is a person's *reaction* to these sensations (or symptoms) resulting from disorder. In the case of pain, this might mean screaming out, retiring to bed, suffering in silence, or pretending it's not happening. These psychological reactions to illness are open to change and this is one of the aims of counselling.

Some tinnitus patients, when they see their doctor, make a very strong demand for a medical cure. Nothing less than the complete elimination of the noises, it seems, will suffice. This poses a dilemma for the doctor. On the one hand, there are always new tests to perform and new drugs to experiment with. On the other hand, the desire for medical treatment may be unrealistic but this message is difficult to get across to unreceptive ears. A doctor might explain the role of psychological and stress factors and point out that drugs or masking can ameliorate the effects of tinnitus. But if the patient regards this as insufficient, there is little to be done except to offer continuing support or discontinue treatment. The doctor will probably offer follow-up appointments to a patient with this attitude, hoping that the problem will improve or that expectations about treatment will change.

A person who is seeking a cure will often go on to explore the many types of alternative medicine now available, such as acupuncture or herbal remedies. My only comment here is that I do not know of any branch of complementary medicine that claims to have success in *eliminating* tinnitus, although relief from the suffering it causes can sometimes be obtained in this way.

Psychological counselling and therapy

Because there is such a sharp division between the physical and mental health services, referral to an expert in the 'mind' might seem to be a bigger and more ominous decision than it really is. I am fortunate that I work in a clinic where several professional groups work alongside the doctors, but this is not a very common practice as far as psychological counselling is concerned.

The mental distress that tinnitus causes is not especially mysterious or the outcome of deep subconscious motives. However, if you are referred to a therapist who knows little about tinnitus and attempts to interpret its deep significance you might feel justifiably that this is not what you are looking for. Although I have come across examples of this sort, it is fortunately a rare occurrence. What is needed, and this is also rare, is a therapist who knows the subject of tinnitus and immediately recognizes what you are talking about. A trained therapist or counsellor does not need additional skills so much as a general familiarity with tinnitus and its effects. This is important because I often find during counselling that my client has not fully absorbed the medical facts already conveyed in the medical consultation. There is usually additional information to give as well. A booklet comes in handy here to present some basic facts and explain the rationale of the psychological approach.

In the assessments I routinely make prior to offering a course of therapy, I consider the following three questions:

- Is extended counselling really necessary?
- Does my client have an adequate understanding of the causes of his or her predicament and the 'labels' that are being applied?
- Is tinnitus really the main problem?

Let me discuss each of these questions in turn.

'Leaving well alone'

Counselling is one form of paying attention to tinnitus. Discussing tinnitus and thinking of it as an important problem can make it more noticeable. Monitoring tinnitus from week to week in a diary can also be counter-productive. I have noticed that some

clients returning for their follow-up appointments become more
bothered by their noises a few days in advance of seeing me. For
these sorts of reasons, and if I believe that there are signs of tolerance developing, I often give the advice 'to leave well alone'. This
is a fine judgement, but I have found that after being reassured
about their concerns, many of the people I interview come to this
conclusion themselves. Distress caused by tinnitus is likely to
decline of its own accord and this can be checked out at a later
date.

'Labelling yourself or being labelled'

Chance events are often seen to be the result of your own doing
even when it is difficult to see how you *could* be responsible for
them. The result is self-blame and deprecatory self-labelling. Tinnitus strikes 'at random' but you might still feel in some way responsible for it and guilty for being unable to cope 'as well as you
should'. You have no grounds for blaming yourself in this way
except in the unlikely event that you wilfully exposed yourself
to very loud sounds or consumed large quantities of aspirin knowing it to make your noises louder! It would be unusual if you were
aware of the damage being done to your ears at the time it was
occurring and so there is no reason to believe that you have
brought the problem on yourself. It is disconcerting, therefore,
to hear occasionally of someone who has been blamed by a 'therapist' for their noises, for example, being told that the noises are
the result of 'pent up anger'.

There is perhaps a better case for saying that you are partly
responsible for the emotional effects of tinnitus.

However, taking responsibility for *that* does not mean taking
on all kinds of labels such as being 'weak', 'neurotic' or 'hysteri-
cal'. A tendency to label yourself in this way is understandable,
and family members or doctors may have reinforced the idea.
Perhaps because tinnitus is invisible and apparently harmless, it
is not surprising that labelling yourself or being labelled in a negative way are so common. I must stress that *it is quite normal* for
noises to be distressing. This can be understood by anyone who
has suffered from external noise.

'Tinnitus not the main problem'

Being such an obvious irritant, tinnitus could become a convenient
scapegoat for all your problems. In reality, life is not so simple

that tinnitus can be held generally responsible for all that is amiss. Certainly, tinnitus *is* a source of annoyance but most people have other sources of frustration, disappointment or worry as well. It may be difficult to pinpoint the causes of the latter and so tinnitus can come in as a convenient explanation.

There are several ways in which tinnitus combines with other problems. In the simplest, it's just an additional worry but perhaps the one that tips the balance so that you feel that you are not coping at all. In other cases, there is a snowball effect; tinnitus magnifies some pre-existing problem or, because of some pre-existing circumstances, tinnitus is much more significant.

Let me give a few examples. The process of attending to the noises is influenced by the mood you are in. In a low mood you are more distractable and morbid thoughts are more likely to arise. When you are already depressed or anxious for other reasons, it will therefore be more difficult to 'switch off' from the noises. Tinnitus is irritating; your mood deteriorates; you have more worrying and depressing thoughts about it; and a vicious cycle sets in. To give another example, the onset of tinnitus may have special significance because a relative has had the same problem and developed deafness as well. Naturally you wonder if this is going to be your fate as well.

In these circumstances, a problem that seems unrelated to tinnitus might be the best one to tackle in counselling. It is only after a lengthy assessment that the wisdom of this approach becomes apparent. When other problems are dealt with successfully, a person starts to feel more confident all round and the noises can lose much of their importance.

Final remarks

I will be describing therapeutic techniques in subsequent chapters. Here, I want to add a few final remarks on seeking help.

You may consider yourself the kind of person who copes well with stress. Remember, however, that tinnitus is different from most other problems. You cannot do much about it in an active forthright manner. This approach might work well with *external* noise pollution when an angry and well-directed complaint might get the source of noise removed. But in the case of *internal* noise pollution anger is counter-productive. You will not be able to call in anyone to fix the problem. As an active, coping type of person you might be successful in getting to see your local tinnitus expert but you will not necessarily want to take the advice offered to slow down and learn to relax. To put matters simply, it is important to be flexible when coping with stress and not to assume that tinnitus is just like any other problem.

I have three main psychological strategies to offer. The first, mentioned above, is to deal with problems that are indirectly related to tinnitus. The second is to dislodge the attitudes and beliefs that *prevent* the acceptance of tinnitus and therefore the natural development of tolerance. This is where cognitive therapy techniques come into their own. The third strategy is to help you control your emotional reaction to stressors (including your noises) so that you learn *not* to respond when the noises are annoying. The first step in this approach is to identify the stress trigger points in your life and the tinnitus diary is useful in this respect. Relaxation and other methods are used for stress reduction.

Counselling and therapy of the kind I am describing are not widely available. There are of course many skilled therapists around but some of them shy away from tinnitus thinking it requires special skills. There is some truth in this but the knowledge or skill deficit could easily be rectified by a little reading and by taking the plunge and seeing a few clients with tinnitus.

Counselling and relaxation training is often available from the staff in a tinnitus clinic. Besides doctors, there are audiological scientists, technicians, hearing therapists and sometimes lay counsellors who are there to listen to your difficulties. Referral to a clinical psychologist, psychiatrist or social worker is usually possible. Beyond the network surrounding the tinnitus clinic, there are likely to be clinical psychologists in your locality to whom you can be referred. Classess in relaxation, meditation, and yoga are often available in Adult Education Colleges or Community Centres. You might find that attending a class of this sort or joining a self-help tinnitus group (see Chapter 11) is sufficient for your needs.

8
Cognitive therapy techniques

In Chapters 5 and 6 I attempted to show the link between paying attention to the noises and the beliefs you hold about them. You may have found the arguments convincing but still feel unable to put 'acceptance' into practice because you may feel that some of your beliefs about tinnitus are true or too difficult to change. In this chapter I intend to explore what these beliefs might be (you are not necessarily aware of them) and how you can be helped to change them if you are inclined to do so.

It is essential in therapy to lend yourself to persuasion. However, you may hold your beliefs with such conviction that they are unassailable by any methods I suggest here. For example, if you firmly believe that the only acceptable solution to tinnitus is the complete elimination of the noises, then there is little room for persuasion. A therapist can only hope to be successful when you are open to an alternative point of view. I hope that I will touch on certain beliefs that you would like to be argued out of, simply because giving them up would diminish your distress. For example: 'Tinnitus means I will have to give up work' or 'Tinnitus means I will never be able to enjoy my life again' are beliefs that most people would prefer not to hold.

There are two kinds of belief to consider. First, there are beliefs about the causes of tinnitus, how it is likely to affect you, and what will happen as a result of having tinnitus. Second, there are beliefs about what to do about tinnitus — whether, for example, to change your diet, learn to relax, or join a self-help group. Beliefs about what tinnitus *is* or means to you and beliefs about the best thing to do about it are related but not completely connected. For the moment, I am concerned about what tinnitus *means* to you.

As I explained in Chapter 6, *any* belief that gives tinnitus meaning is likely to slow down the natural development of tolerance. We pay attention to sensations that have some significance for us. We stop paying attention to (ignore) sensations that are repetitious and have no meaning. There are two purposes to the cognitive techniques I describe in this chapter. The first is to help you come to regard tinnitus noises as unworthy of attention because they are predictably familiar and have no meaning. When you can ignore tinnitus completely, the noises might as well not exist. This is the ideal state, and the aim of my psychological approach is to help you along this path as far as possible. The second purpose is to help you become less distressed by the tinnitus even when you hear it.

The methods we have found useful in changing beliefs are based on the cognitive therapies of Aaron Beck and Albert Ellis developed in the United States. In this chapter I give a flavour of what this is all about but do not expect you to come away with the ability to apply these techniques to yourself. They contain a good measure of self-help but an experienced therapist is definitely required for overall guidance. My chief reason for going into as much detail as I do is the fact that many readers are likely to be unfamiliar with them. A few self-help books on the subject are listed in the bibliography at the back of this book.

Cognitive therapy principles

The first principle of cognitive therapy is that thoughts cause feeling. By 'thought' I mean things you say to yourself, images, beliefs, general assumptions about the world, and also certain styles of thinking. Even though it might seem that you cannot help the way you feel or that you are in the grip of emotion, the truth of the matter is that underlying your feeling is a certain way of thinking. The thinking process may be so habitual, so automatic, that you may not even recognize it. The therapist's first task is, therefore, to help reveal to the client the thoughts that underly his or her feelings of distress.

So, in reading these words you might be feeling despondent (*Thought*: this sounds too simple, it won't work for me) or anxious (*Thought*: this sounds too complicated, I won't get the hang of this) or cheerful (*Thought*: perhaps there is some way of lessening the effect of these noises after all). To reveal what you are thinking about tinnitus takes time and effort and this is where much of the skill of a cognitive therapist comes in.

Once the automatic thoughts have been identified the next step is to dispute them and replace them by more positive and constructive ways of thinking. The method of disputation works by showing that the thoughts are based on faulty reasoning. Some thoughts are simply illogical, while others are based on a selective view of the evidence. Some thoughts seem to be factually correct, but on examination it turns out that *feelings* are being taken as facts. For example, tinnitus can be intrusive and can interfere with mental concentration. This is a fact. However, how you *feel* about this loss of concentration depends on how important it is for you to concentrate at a particular time and whether you think that others have noticed your loss of concentration. In reality, it might not be so important that you concentrate well *all* the time. Others may not have noticed your lack of concentration anyway. Furthermore, although I stated that it is a fact that tinnitus can affect mental concentration, it is not true that *all* failures of concentration are due to tinnitus. Therefore, you may mistakenly believe that tinnitus is to blame, when in reality your poor concentration is due to tiredness, worrying thoughts or something else.

I have just been applying some cognitive therapy principles — investigating the thoughts behind feelings and the thoughts behind *those* thoughts. Eventually, we reach a bedrock of core beliefs that a person holds onto tightly. Cognitive therapy was originally developed for people chronically afflicted by depressed and anxious moods. It has been found that in many cases such people have core beliefs that make it very hard to lead a normal life.

Examples of core beliefs are 'I'm nothing unless I am loved', 'There are only winners and losers in life' or 'I can't tolerate being out of control'. There is no special reason to believe that people who are affected by tinnitus hold these kinds of core belief unless, of course, they are very depressed or anxious for reasons other than their tinnitus. Nevertheless, I have found that people who suffer with tinnitus share similar ways of thinking with people who are severely depressed or anxious.

The thoughts are not so firmly held or applied to so many situations. However, in order to highlight what I have been discussing, let us first consider the thinking processes of people in more extreme moods. It is often found that the way of thinking associated with anxiety or depression is set on proving the truth of core beliefs so that they become self-fulfilling prophecies. This results in various kinds of illogical reasoning. Take the core belief 'I can't tolerate being out of control'. The following situations show how reasons might be given to support the core belief and result in certain intense feelings.

Situation/Evidence	Thought/Reasoning	Feeling
My neighbour parked his car in front of my drive	1. He is deliberately making it inconvenient for me because I parked in front of his house yesterday..............	Irritation
	2. What if I can't get the car out in an emergency!......	Anxiety

The first thought is an example of an *arbitrary inference*, arbitrary because there might be some equally good explanation for the evidence (The car might have broken down, the neighbour might have parked temporarily and is about to move it, etc.) The reason that is given, however, is consistent with the main concern of being out of control (for example, unable to drive in and out of the drive at that moment.) The thinking process might proceed further to the second thought that some disaster could happen if driving in and out proved impossible. For example, 'this could be terrible if a member of my family had a serious accident and had to be taken to the hospital at a moment's notice.' This type of thinking is called *catastrophic* because it involves overestimating the chances that something of this kind would happen (or that it would be so bad).

Here is a different situation.

Situation/Evidence	Thought/Reasoning	Feeling
A salesman comes to the door and offers something for sale	All salesmen use tricks of the trade to persuade you into buying things you don't want. I'll *never* buy anything from a door-to-door salesman.......	Anger

Two thinking errors are illustrated here. The concern about control (in this case being manipulated) leads the person to *overgeneralize* about *all* door-to-door salesmen. The fact that some or even most salesmen use unfair methods doesn't mean that *all* do. The second error is called *black and white* thinking. There is no grey area in judgement. Either a thing is all good or all bad. The person says they'll *never* buy from a door-to-door salesman even though it might on some occasion prove convenient to do so.

The following situation illustrates some other styles of illogical reasoning.

Situation/Evidence	Thought/Reasoning	Feeling
Your neighbour brings a gift of some cakes saying that her visitors had cancelled, leaving her with more cakes than she could eat.	Your neighbour is trying to curry favour with you.....	Suspicion

There may be a lot of evidence to support your neighbour's account of her gift. Nevertheless a certain interpretation is put on the evidence which conforms with the core belief about control. So, it might be felt that acceptance of the gift would incur an obligation to return it; an obligation might be seen as a restriction of choice and, therefore, a decrease of control; For example, then it would become more difficult to complain about your neighbour's parking habits?

This imaginary scenario illustrates several biased ways of think-ing. The thought that your neighbour is trying to curry favour could be taken to imply: (a) that you have ignored evidence to the contrary and the facts are made to fit in with your own interpretation (this has been called operating a *mental filter*); (b) that you have made no attempt to find out whether the neigh-bour's account is true (this is *a failure to test reality*); (c) that you have discounted your neighbour's positive gesture towards you (this is called *disqualifying the positive*); (d) that you expect some-thing to happen as a consequence, for example, that your neigh-bour will expect a favour from you when in fact your neighbour doesn't expect anything for her gift (this is called the *fortune-telling error*).

These examples illustrate the kinds of thoughts and their associated errors of thinking which a cognitive therapist will try to uncover. What then follows is a process of disputation. This doesn't mean that therapist and client take on the role of adver-saries. The therapist is trying to help the client not prove him or her wrong. Disputing can take the usual verbal form (see below) or, alternatively, tasks are suggested that require a person to face up to new experiences and therefore make new interpretations of the evidence. Thinking differently follows from *doing* things differently whether it's entertaining a novel train of thought or surprising yourself by acting out of character. One aim of the ther-apist is to help the client learn *how* to learn from experience in just the same way that a scientist has to study the results of an experiment to see if they throw light on his or her theory. In a similar way, the client makes self-observations and attempts to become aware of automatic thoughts, recognizing their existence and noting them down. Ways of disputing them are thought up with the help of the therapist. Inconsistencies between what the client thinks and feels, and how they act, are also examined.

The therapist encourages a reconsideration of the validity of the client's beliefs by putting the following sorts of questions:

'What evidence do you have to support your thoughts?'
'What evidence do you have against your thoughts?'
'What alternative views are there?'
'How would someone else view this situation?'
'What is the effect of thinking the way you do?'

'Does it help you or hinder you from getting what you want?'

'Are you thinking in all-or nothing terms?'

'Are you concentrating on your weaknesses and forgetting your strengths?'

'Are you blaming yourself for something which is not your fault?'

'Are you expecting yourself to be perfect?'

'Are you using a double standard — how would you view someone else in your situation?'

'Are you over-estimating the chances of disaster?'

'Are you using a crystal ball to read the future?'

'Are you fretting about the way things ought to be instead of accepting and dealing with them as they come?'

'What can you do to test out the truth of your thoughts?'

The kind of thoughts that go with being emotionally upset often have an all-or-nothing ring about them. They imply that something is 'always', 'forever', or 'never' true. They imply that the thinker 'need', 'should', 'must', or 'can't' do something. The thought allows for no alternative. The therapist might point out that this is a rigid way of viewing matters, but will not suggest that there is any other right way of doing so. The therapist is more likely to think up a menu of alternatives and invite the client to entertain each in turn to see where it leads and whether it feels right.

There is much more to cognitive therapy than I can hope to explain here, so I will now go on to consider tinnitus and some typical thoughts and feelings which may accompany it.

The situations that trigger thoughts about tinnitus include, of course, the presence of noises. Your thoughts about tinnitus are likely to occur at particular times — for example, when the noises are louder, when a new noise appears or when listening to other people is difficult. I have grouped some common feelings and their associated thoughts below.

Feeling: anger, irritation, blame
Possible thoughts:

'I'm not going to put up with it.'

'I'm not going to let these noises beat me.'

'The doctors should come up with a cure for this.'

'My family ought to realize how much this affects me.'

'Dr.......... is responsible for this. I shouldn't have had that test.'

Feeling: resentment, bitterness, persecution
Possible thoughts:
    'If my employers had provided ear defenders I wouldn't have this problem.'
    'It's unfair that a young person like myself should get these noises.'
    'It's unfair that when you get older something like this comes along to spoil your retirement.'
    'I'm not the sort of person to be affected by illness; I can't accept this.'

Feeling: fear, anxiety, worry
Possible thoughts:
    'Suppose the noises get louder.'
    'Suppose I go completely deaf.'
    'Will I be able to cope with this forever?'
    'I could end up financially ruined.'
    'Suppose there is a tumour growing in my head.'

Feeling: helpless, depressed, pessimistic
Possible thoughts:
    'It will be dreadful if these noises never go away.'
    'I can't imagine coping with these noises forever.'
    'Life will not be worth living if these noises continue.'

In a moment I will suggest ways in which these thoughts can be disputed. The purpose of the challenging process is not to prove that you are muddle-headed and that you shouldn't be having these thoughts. The purpose is to see if these thoughts are true or not. In my view, having thoughts that are untrue and also distressing serves no real purpose and prolongs suffering.

In my experience a more philosophical attitude towards the noises leads to increasing tolerance, and the analytical approach of cognitive therapy can help you to achieve this.

What I mean by taking a philosophical attitude is that when your attention is drawn to the noise, you merely note this in the same way that a passing car is noted; an attempt is made to continue with what you are doing. In contrast, engaging in the automatic thoughts listed above entails getting 'worked-up' about the noises. There is an emotional reaction, sometimes accompanied by a gesture, curse or complaint. It is not unusual to find sufferers who literally bang or slap their ears. A vicious cycle of distress and attention to the noises develops. One way to break into this cycle is to observe the negative thoughts and write them down on a card. Against each thought is stated a positive and constructive challenge. Below, I offer you an example of the way a therapist might help a client to reveal negative thoughts and come up with a more positive outlook. The example is fictional and it may not feel right for you. Nevertheless, it should give some idea of the process at work and help you to generate your own challenges. The thoughts and challenges can be written on a card and kept in a pocket as a reminder as needed.

One of the most common thoughts is that things will get worse in the future. This is the 'dreadfulizing' process so common in worry. Let us consider the fear that tinnitus will get worse in some way.

Fictional dialogue between therapist (T) and client (C)

T   What is your evidence that the noises will get worse?
C   Well they're louder now than they used to be
T   What is your evidence that they will get still louder?
C   I feel they might get louder.
T   Feeling that something will happen doesn't mean that it will. In fact, in the majority of cases the loudness of tinnitus stays about the same and doesn't get louder.
C   Yes, but I still worry that it might get louder because it sometimes does get louder.
T   The fact that the noises are *sometimes* louder doesn't mean that they will *remain* louder. What would be so bad if they did get louder?
C   I couldn't cope with it.
T   What is your evidence that you couldn't cope?
C   When it gets louder now I'm quite useless, unable to do anything.
T   You said that the noises have already got louder. Have you managed to cope with this increase?
C   Well...Yes. But I'm still back to square one when it's really loud.
T   You mean you feel just as badly as when this problem first started to trouble you?

C   Well not exactly but I'm hopeless when it's loud.

T   So there has been some general improvement but there are bad patches?

C   Yes.

T   In these bad patches you said you feel 'quite useless, unable to do anything'. Can you describe to me what you mean?

C   I just stay in bed and have the radio on loud to drown out the noises.

T   So there is something you can do — listen to the radio. Do you think there is anything else you could do?

C   Well I suppose I feel so depressed I don't want to do anything.

T   So things are not so black and white as you painted. Not wanting to do something is not quite the same as being unable to do something, is it? Did you ever get depressed and lie around before these noises started?

C   Well I suppose I did sometimes but not as much as now.

T   So you get more depressed now. Why do you think that is?

C   The tinnitus is much worse, it really depresses me.

T   Tinnitus can be a lot more troublesome when you're feeling low because you have little interest in things that would distract you. I think it's important to consider whether there might be other reasons for your feelings of depression. We could then focus on these other reasons and then if we were successful the noises would be less bothersome. What do you think about that?

C   Well, I think it's thinking about tinnitus that depresses me. I see myself going downhill.

T   You have made an important point. Perhaps it's imagining the consequences of tinnitus that depresses you rather than the way it affects you here and now. Just to recap on our discussion, we seem to have reached the following conclusions. First, the fact that the noises *might* get louder doesn't mean that they will. Second, that you're generally less distressed now than you once were, even though the noises have, as you say, got louder. So you have coped with the noises getting louder already. Third, that when the noises are loud you are not completely useless and unable to do anything. In fact we have yet to find out what you are really capable of doing despite the noises. Fourth, there may be reasons other than the noises for your feeling depressed right now. And, as you say, it's what you think about the tinnitus that depresses you — we will have to go into these thoughts to see if they are justified.

This is a contrived dialogue devised to illustrate just a few of the ways in which automatic negative thoughts can be disputed (I hope you can pick out the thoughts and the challenges.) The session would probably be followed up by some suggested exercises designed to discover what the client was capable of doing when the noises were loud (for example, learning to type on a noisy typewriter producing both a distracting and a masking effect.) This dialogue might sound a little like a cross-examination. If so, this is not intended. One way to avoid getting into this trap is to ask the client to take on the therapist's role and do the challenging while the therapist plays the client. In this way, the client learns to use the challenges on him or herself because in this 'reverse role-playing' method the client is arguing against his/her own beliefs. It is useful to have a list of the possible challenges available so that the client is prompted to use them rather than rely purely on memory. If the client gets stuck, the therapist can point out some of the challenges that might work.

Analysing your irrational thoughts and disputing them

On each occasion that the noises affect you emotionally, it is useful to make a note under four headings which can be abbreviated to ABCD. A is the Activating event; B stands for Beliefs; C refers to the Consequences (on your feelings and actions); D stands for Dispute. To start with, only C, the feelings to which tinnitus gives rise will be obvious. You will notice, however, that they are more likely to arise in certain situations as the following example illustrates:

Activating Event	Belief	Consequences	Dispute
It has been difficult to mix with people for some time. You go out to dinner and come back early because of the noises.		You feel dispirited and hopeless about the future	

Now ask yourself what beliefs or thoughts are causing your emotional response here. How are you interpreting this situation and your action of returning home? What does it mean to you? Perhaps the thought is something like 'Socializing is a waste of time' or 'It was difficult enough tonight; how will it be in a few years time?' It is instructive to take this process of analysis further. 'Why was socializing a waste of time?' This question might prompt the next thought: 'The babble of voices set my noises off. I couldn't think straight. I was left out of the conversation.' As a therapist, I have found that by questioning further and further in this way, one can reveal fundamental beliefs such as 'Others think I'm stupid'. You may have some difficulty reaching these core beliefs without the assistance of a therapist. It is unpleasant to admit to them and, in any case, they may be so hidden as to lie outside your reach. The more firmly held and wrongly founded your beliefs the more they are likely to affect you emotionally.

The next stage is to dispute your thoughts using the challenges listed earlier. The form of words that successfully disputes the thought is written down under D. For example 'Socializing is a waste of time' could be regarded as black and white thinking and disputed as follows: 'I didn't enjoy the evening as much as in the past but that doesn't mean that I didn't enjoy it all. There were moments I enjoyed and these made the evening worthwhile.' Again, you could dispute the thought that you couldn't think straight and were left out of the conversation by asking 'What is the evidence?', and seek feedback to test the truth of your belief. Do you remember any of the conversation? Did others think you made no conversation? After sifting the evidence, you might write down under D 'Nobody told me I didn't make sense when I asked them later. I didn't say as much as I wanted to but everyone appreciated my presence.

Here are some typical ABCD's to help you with your self-analysis.

A	B	C	D
The noises are louder than usual.	There must be a serious cause for such a loud noise (like a tumour).	I feel anxious	Tests have revealed nothing. I have no other symptoms to indicate a tumour. I have had the noises for five years and something like a tumour would have shown up long before now.

A	B	C	D
You read an article that suggests that in the forseeable future a cure for tinnitus will not be found.	It's unfair that my retirement has been spoiled by these noises. There ought to be a cure.	I feel bitter.	Perhaps I don't have a right to stay completely healthy until I die. In fact, compared to my friends, I am pretty healthy. In any case, why do I assume that I won't be able to come to terms with this? It doesn't help to think this way.

A	B	C	D
Your tinnitus has got louder and stayed that way for a week.	It's going to stay like this forever. I won't be able to cope.	This is dreadful, I despair.	It's been loud before — there's no reason why it won't ease off as it did in the past. How do I know I won't be able to cope if it stays louder? There are times that I cope well when it's loud. I am discounting my strengths and dwelling on my weaknesses.

Cognitive therapy in groups

Instead of using cognitive techniques in one-to-one therapy, the same methods can be applied to a group of clients who share the problem of tinnitus. We have generally worked on the basis of seven participants and two therapists. The group meets weekly for two hours on six occasions. Usually, the group is extended for another six sessions to reinforce what has been learned. There are several advantages to group therapy. The participants share a common problem and can support each other. They quickly learn that their troubles are not unique. At the same time, they learn that there are marked differences in the way that people can be affected. This may come as a surprise and suggest to them that their own response is not an inevitable consequence of tinnitus.

The therapists demonstrate how to dispute beliefs before the participants are asked to try it for themselves. Some members of the group are helped rapidly. This gives the other participants faith in the method. Another very important source of inspiration comes from members of previous groups who have already benefited from therapy. We are grateful to several ex-clients who come along on one occasion to recount their experience of coping with tinnitus. They are far more convincing than we can ever be in demonstrating that change is possible.

Availability of cognitive therapy

It is only in the last 5-10 years that cognitive techniques have become widely used. The opportunities for therapists to train in these methods is still rather limited. Consequently, cognitive therapy is not readily available. It is a method that is still in the research and evaluation stage as far as tinnitus is concerned, and so until it has been proved to meet its initial promise the situation is unlikely to change. Our own research, as yet unpublished, indicates that around 45 per cent of the participants in group cognitive therapy benefit considerably.

9
Relaxation and self-suggestion

'Just relax' is not always a welcome piece of advice; if you have a persistently annoying noise you may wish heartily that you could follow it. A common way of coping with tinnitus is not to relax but to do the opposite and become busier and busier. By directing your attention outwardly, an inward dwelling on the noises is avoided.

However, learning how to relax deeply can be a useful way to counteract an annoying tinnitus. If you take this path, you should have a serious intention to practise relaxation every day and to apply it at times of stress. Half-measures are unlikely to yield benefit. Published research shows that about 30-40 per cent of people whose tinnitus has distressed them for some years can expect to feel less annoyed and less disturbed by it if they practise and apply relaxation for two to three months. It is not yet clear why relaxation produces these benefits but, having researched the method myself, I believe that it can help in at least three ways:

1. *An overactive mind and body.* Learning to relax helps the kind of person who deals with stressful situations 'head on' and ends up filling every spare moment of the day — a lifestyle that may have developed in response to head noises or may have been part of a person's character beforehand. If you feel uncomfortable when required to wait patiently or find it impossible just to sit in a quiet room, then learning to relax should provide a powerful antidote. It is what you least like doing and, therefore, on the assumption that 'the medicine should be distasteful', what you really need. Your active lifestyle may have served you well in the past but tinnitus can tip a positive, action-oriented approach into a negative, frenetic one. Learning to relax means achieving quiet repose when

you need it — especially when trying to get off to sleep or to go back to sleep when woken up in the night (see later under 'Insomnia').

2. *Avoiding your noises.* It might seem impossible to avoid a noise in your head, but feeling *compelled* to engage in distracting activity is a form of avoidance. You are avoiding having to listen to your noises. It is paradoxical but true that in order to ignore the noises you have to listen to them. Ignoring is the end-result of over-familiarization — but this is only one arm of a two-pronged strategy. It is also important to deal with the 'unfinished business' which I discussed in chapters 5 and 6. Listening to tinnitus is best done in a state of relaxation when you can more easily dismiss negative thoughts and control the temptation to tense up, or even curse.

3. *Negative images of tinnitus.* Relaxation provides the right mental state in which to experiment with techniques for changing your *image* of tinnitus. By an image, I mean your interpretation or perception of the noises. This might be positive (for example, the soothing tinkle of a stream) or negative (for example, a piercing howl). Your image of tinnitus and even its loudness are to some extent under your control. Techniques for modifying images will be described later.

Learning to relax

It is important first of all to understand what you are trying to achieve by learning to relax. As I have hinted, relaxation can be of greater value to you than simply learning how to flop down in a heap on a bed. At its most successful, teaching yourself to relax will help you to feel tranquil when it is appropriate to do so, allowing you to switch your attention at will from the noises to whatever else you are doing. As a deliberate strategy for dealing with stress, it will help you to cope calmly without excessive muscular and mental effort.

Secondly, choose a method and practise it so that you begin to recognize when you are feeling tense and/or mentally over-charged and when you are feeling calm and mentally at peace. It is difficult to define relaxation in a positive sense but you will learn to recognize the state as you practise the exercise. You will go into it more quickly and more deeply as time goes on. It has been described as a floating sensation. You are awake with a clear mind — in fact images take on a vivid, dream-like quality. Although you are not sleepy, relaxation helps you to pass into a state of sleep more easily.

There are several methods to help you learn to relax. One method is to learn the difference between muscle tension and relaxation by alternately tensing and relaxing muscle groups in different parts of the body. Other methods focus on breathing, or on self-suggestions of warmth and heaviness, or on conjuring up pleasant and relaxing mental images. What they all have in common is the requirement to sit or lie comfortably without external distraction. With your eyes closed your attention is fully on the technique you are following. This may involve listening to repeated instructions given in a low monotonous voice while at the same time you are concentrating on your immediate feelings and sensations. 'Busy thinking' is left far behind as you concentrate on a single thought, image or sensation. The effect is to produce both mental and bodily calmness. Your body is likely to feel heavy and limp and your breathing will be slow and gentle.

I will not at this point describe the various methods of relaxation training. You can find detailed descriptions of the techniques in paperback books on the subject (see Bibliography). However, there are a few points worth bearing in mind. First, it is easier to learn relaxation when you are guided by an experienced therapist. Later you can practise with an audiotape (these are also commercially available) and eventually dispense with these aids altogether.

The advantage of starting with a therapist, or in a class run by an expert, is that you are more likely to make rapid progress initially. In this way you will avoid the discouragement that could arise if your practise by yourself. You are also more likely to keep up your exercises — which should be followed once or twice a day for about twenty minutes.

Second, the actual method you use is probably not that important as long as you like it. If you have any joint or muscle problems you should avoid the muscle tensing/ relaxing method. Strenuous tensing is not, in any case, necessary. Mental calmness can also be achieved by the method of autogenic training or through transcendental meditation. If you have a more physical orientation, you may prefer Yoga, T'ai Ch'i, or the Alexander Technique.

Third, for some people to let go and relax is itself unpleasant.

Letting go may allow thoughts to emerge that you would rather suppress. Relaxation may produce sensations that are unfamiliar to you, as if you are losing control of your body, exposed and vulnerable. You might even find tears welling up in your eyes and worry about reacting in this way. These effects should not be long-lasting and so it is worth persisting. If they continue to concern you, seek professional advice.

Fourth, having learned 'passive relaxation' you should go on to apply it 'actively' as a technique for dealing with stressful situations, and even to adopt it as part of your daily philosophy (see under Active Relaxation).

Lastly, if you have a severe hearing loss, a relaxation technique that involves listening to tape-recorded instructions will be a strain at best and impossible at worst. With just a few minor modifications to technique, live relaxation classes can be run successfully for people who are deaf. In fact, many of the techniques I have mentioned involve simple instructions which can be committed to memory for practice at home. Watching a demonstration of the exercises is helpful. A therapist can prompt a sequence of instructions by using a system of tactile or visual signals.

The techniques of biofeedback and hypnosis have also been used in treating tinnitus psychologically. For this reason I will briefly describe them and explain how their application fits in with what I have said so far.

Biofeedback

Biofeedback catches the imagination because it promises a way of controlling bodily states without the use of drugs. Enthusiasm for the method, together with the marketing efforts of manufacturers of cheap biofeedback instruments, has produced a high level of public awareness.

Very simply, biofeedback allows the active, conscious mind to respond to events in our body of which we are normally unaware. In fact, for events in the brain (which can be detected in the form of the electroencephalogram or EEG), there is no natural way of sensing their presence at all. One of the most popular devices feeds back information about the degree of sweating in the palm of the hand. The amount of sweat is detected electronically and converted to a signal such as a buzzing sound. This is the feedback signal of the bodily response and the sound changes in pitch according to the degree of sweating. It is the task of the person wearing the device to control the direction of change of the signal — for example, to lower the pitch of the buzzing sound. The important thing is to *achieve* this result, though the way you do it may remain a mystery.

It is not known what bodily response produces tinnitus and so, strictly speaking, biofeedback techniques cannot be applied. However, the chief value of biofeedback in coping with tinnitus is to learn control of the bodily responses associated with emotional (stress) reactions. For example, a high heart rate, emotional sweating, and muscle tension, can be reduced in this way. There is no evidence that for people with tinnitus, biofeedback has any special advantage over other methods of learning to relax. However, you might find that this method suits you. Muscle tension biofeedback is helpful if the muscles of the head, neck, or jaw are especially tense. It is advisable to try out the technique before committing yourself to the expense of an instrument or a course of therapy.

Hypnosis

Hypnosis is an altered state of awareness which has much in common with relaxation and is perhaps an extension of it. In a hypnotic trance, a person is more receptive to the voice of the therapist and the messages the voice conveys. Hypnotists have several techniques at their disposal for inducing a heightened susceptibility to their suggestions. These include asking the client to adopt a tiring posture (eyes rolled back, arms raised, etc.) and then suggesting the feelings of fatigue that inevitably follow. Whatever it is, becoming 'hypnotized' does not of itself achieve anything. Hypnotists who use the technique therapeutically are called hypnotherapists. Their success depends on what methods are applied in the hypnotic state and, for tinnitus, these are broadly the same as the ones that I describe below for use during relaxation.

The results of one recent trial of hypnotherapy are interesting because they show what can and cannot be achieved with this method where tinnitus is concerned. Besides learning to relax, it was suggested to the participants in the study that the loudness of the noises would reduce and that they would in fact cease. These suggestions were conveyed in the form of an image selected by the participant, for example, unplugging a connection on an old-fashioned telephone switchboard. In only *one* case out of four-teen did the noises seem to get quieter at the end of therapy. Nevertheless, one third of the participants said that they were less annoyed by their noises and tolerated them better. Perhaps it was the relaxation component or the concentrated attention on the noises that helped in this respect. The author of the report, an experienced hypnotherapist, found it puzzling that, in con-trast to pain where a total anaesthesia can be produced in a good hypnotic subject, tinnitus cannot be switched off in the same way.

Auto-hypnosis (self-hypnosis)

Successful hypnosis is really self-hypnosis. During the induction procedure you allow *yourself* to follow the suggestions of the hyp-notherapist and then take them away from the session as self-instructions. For example, if the therapist suggests to you that you will feel relaxed when you say the word 'relax', this is really an instruction to yourself. Strictly speaking, auto-hypnosis means put-ting yourself into trance but the purpose of the trance is to respond more promptly and with a clear and concentrated mind to your own self-suggestions.

Some hypnotherapists make an audio recording of their sessions so that the client can take it away to listen to at home. If for one reason or another the tape is ineffective, modifications to the induction can be recorded in a future session. The initial pur-pose of home-practice is to achieve deep relaxation. Later on, instructions for specific problems are added to the tape. The tape ends with a statement of the following kind: 'In a few moments you will open your eyes and feel refreshed...feeling good...alert...so alive.' Of course, this is omitted when the purpose of the tape is to promote sleep!

If you can ill-afford hypnotherapy (and it is advisable to choose someone reputable) there are do-it-yourself guides which show you how to make your own self-induction tapes (see Bibliogra-phy). Examples of scripts are given for individual problems, includ-ing tinnitus. My experience of this form of self-help is limited so I cannot comment on its effectiveness.

The attainment of a deeply relaxed state or hypnotic trance is the means rather than the end of therapy. It is the means, first, to the deliberate use of relaxation to cope with stress (active or applied relaxation) and, second, to developing and rehearsing helpful self-instructions and mental images. Let us take each of these applications in turn.

Active (applied) relaxation

Having learned to relax 'passively' in your comfortable chair or in a lying position, you can go on to extend this skill so that it becomes of greater use to you in stressful situations. Many day-to-day activities are performed better, with less cost to you, in a relaxed frame of mind. Driving is an obvious example. The hunched shoulders, white knuckles on steering wheel, and grimacing face, are a standard for cartoonists. This extreme is easy to recognize, especially in others. It is rather more difficult to detect milder versions of this reaction in yourself.

However, before you can *apply* relaxation, you must know *when* to apply it — which means increasing your awareness of your own tense bodily reactions. It is also important to detect these early on before they become so overwhelmingly strong that no amount of applied relaxation will prove effective. You can learn to become more aware by stopping yourself at various points in the day and noting whether you are exerting more energy, physical or emotional, than is strictly necessary. For example, occasionally noting down the tension you feel in the facial muscles can be instructive and also indicative of your real mood.

The eventual aim is to progress towards a change in the way all activities are approached. Some therapists see this as developing into a general philosophy of 'flowing with life problems'. Stated very bluntly, without the elaboration it deserves, this philosophy can be expressed as follows:

● To fully accept that life inevitably throws up problems, and everyday something will happen that we do not like.
● To calmly accept undesirable events and to ask oneself whether or not they can be changed.
● To realize deeply that many things cannot be changed. Things said or done cannot be unsaid or undone. To accept that our influence over the behaviour of others is often very limited.
● To recognize that a situation can often be improved by thinking ahead, by adopting a more accepting attitude

to oneself and others, and by always looking at the potential for a positive outcome of a situation instead of its negative aspects.

Applying this philosophy of 'flowing with the problem' to tinnitus (and the hearing loss that often accompanies it) means accepting that you have a handicap, that you will not always hear 100 per cent of what is being said, that the effort required to concentrate will not always be worthwhile, that you will not always enjoy every theatre performance you attend, and so on. Reflecting on this, you will probably acknowledge that this state of affairs existed (at least to some degree) before tinnitus ever became a problem for you.

Relaxing on cue
Keeping this practical wisdom in mind as something to aim for, you might like to try initially some specific techniques for learning to relax on cue. The idea is to take a word or phrase or mental image and pair it with the relaxation you achieve when circumstances are ideal, that is, during your daily passive relaxation exercises. One method is to say the word 'relax' when you breathe out, making the most of the natural relaxation of tension that occurs at this moment. When applying this technique at a moment of stress, you take a breath, hold it briefly while tensing, and then release the breath upon relaxing the tension. Cue words that people have found helpful are 'easy', 'peace', and 'lots of time'.

Instead of words, visual images can be paired with relaxation. The image should be one that helps to induce a feeling of calmness in you, such as a favourite place or a beach scene. The image is called to mind at moments of irritation, nervousness or frustration. You attempt to relax away these thoughts and feelings, while continuing with the task in hand. As a first step in extending your relaxation skill, it is a good idea to apply relaxation to such simple activities as walking, or sitting in an upright chair.

Tinnitus may be present continuously but this is not to say that your reaction to it is unvarying. The moments of tension may occur when hearing or concentration are impaired, when tiredness diminishes your effors to concentrate, or when the noises are especially noticeable in quiet surroundings. It is important to get to know what situations bring out your emotional reactions (see Chapter 4 on keeping a diary). You will then be prepared to

put relaxation into practice and catch yourself reacting emotionally before tension gets a hold on you.

Image rehearsal

Rather than begin with the more difficult task of applying relaxation in real-life, you can start by rehearsing the skill in imagination. First, list the situations that distress you from the least to
the most bothersome. Take the least bothersome first and obtain
a vivid image of it for about 10-20 seconds before deliberately
switching to relaxing. Continue with this image until you can easily
master your negative emotional response to it. Then take the next
situation from the list and repeat.

Switching attention

Just listening to the tinnitus noise may bother you. In this case,
use part of your relaxation exercise to alternate between listening
intently to your noises and switching back to achieve deep relaxation. It is helpful to have another sound to focus on when switching back. This could be the sound of tape-recorded suggestions
for relaxation, relaxing music, or simply the background environmental sounds that are always present. If you have a good capacity for mental imagery, a mental picture of your favourite place
may hold your attention better than an external sound.

Modifying your perception of tinnitus

You may have noticed that the same recording of a piece of music
is enjoyable at one time and disagreeable at another. This illustrates the varying nature of your perception of sound sensations,
even though they are sent out in an identical way by your audio
equipment. If this is so, perhaps your tinnitus could be perceived
differently? It is certainly the case that a few people *like* their tinnitus and would feel lost without it. How is this possible?

A subtle change in perception may occur when tinnitus first
begins. You may assume automatically that the noise is external
— that it is the rumble of lorries or a quirk of the plumbing system. Only later do you realize that the noises originate within
your body because they follow you around. The noises are then
perceived as more sinister; they are seen as less controllable and
possibly as signifying a serious medical disorder.

When you have reached the point that relaxation comes quickly and easily you can begin to experiment with the way you perceive your noises. As a test of whether this is likely to work for you, place an old ticking clock nearby during your relaxation practice. Listen to the tick and imagine:

> The mechanism causing the tick...gear wheels...ratchets... springs...see the mechanism in your mind's eye...see it growing in size so that the tick gets louder...and louder... steel against steel...clanking and crashing...ratchets the size of big hammers...the tick deafening you...the vibrations passing through your body...the clock engulfing you... surrounded now by the mechanism of a huge clock.

> Now imagine the reverse process. You escape from the clock... You see it before you...the tick gets quieter as you move away...the mechanism is contracting...it's getting smaller...receding into the distance...it's so small and delicate...it's hard to imagine how it works...the tick is barely audible.

This exercise demonstrates (if it works at all) that your perception of sound is modifiable. It is now up to you to experiment with images that help you to modify your perception of your own noises. Here are some suggestions:

Externalizing images

Tinnitus is rarely perceived as if coming from outside the head. It is usually heard 'in the head' or 'in the ear'. We think of our minds as being in our heads (even though the mind doesn't really have a physical location) and so noises 'in the head' represent an intrusion into our most personal space. It is therefore an advantage, if at all possible, to externalize your perception of the noise. For example, your pulsating noise is *not* in your head; you are on an ocean cruiser, and you hear the comforting throb of the ship's engines, lulling you to sleep as you relax on deck.

Distancing images

Images can be developed to help you externalize by putting a distance between yourself and the noise. For example: (1) The noise

is a fog, enveloping you; you swim upwards, out of it, into the
sunshine. (2) You descend with the noise in an elevator. You ascend
again, leaving the noise behind you.

Positive images

The example of the ship's engines illustrates another principle.
The noise is perceived as part of a pleasant scene. The whistle
in your ear is really the rustle of autumn leaves or the sound of
telegraph wires vibrating in a summer breeze. The image you
choose depends on your memories and the associations they call
forth. The closer the match between your modified image and
the quality of the tinnitus sound the better.

Diminishing images

Here you exert control over the image. For example: (1) The noise
is emitted from a machine which you control with a lever: as you
pull the lever the sound decreases. (2) The noise is the sound of
gas escaping from a cylinder: slowly, you turn off the valve and
with it the escaping gas.

The images you choose to rehearse during your relaxation exercises are likely to be quite special to you. You may need several
so that you can switch from one to the other. Experiments with
imagery will be most successful after you have acquired the ability to relax deeply. I cannot promise you that they will be effective. The techniques have not been systematically evaluated.
However, they have certainly worked for *some* individuals, as
numerous reports in the technical literature testify.

Researchers in New York have described a surprisingly simple
method which is similar to image modification. By careful measurement, they find an external sound that exactly matches the
pitch and loudness of their client's tinnitus. During the procedure, the intensity of the external sound is lowered in very small
steps. The task for the client is to concentrate on reducing the
loudness of his or her own noise until it matches the external
sound. At this point, the external sound is reduced again and
the process is repeated. Again, all that we can say about this
method is that for *some* people who have tried it, tinnitus became
less annoying. In one case, the noise disappeared for a number
of hours.

Insomnia

Just about a half of the people who attend tinnitus clinics have difficulty getting to sleep, or find themselves waking frequently in the night. In one survey of the British population, one in twenty claimed that tinnitus was responsible for spoiling their sleep.

Drug treatment of insomnia can lead to dependence on sleeping tablets and this is of concern to some people with tinnitus. Sleep is often severely affected when tinnitus begins and it is not unreasonable to turn to hypnotic drugs at this time. However, if sleeplessness is still a problem several months later, it is worth considering an alternative to night sedation.

Sleep disturbance can be a sign of depression but, of course, insomnia can also occur in the absence of depression. The most common form of sleeplessness associated with depression is that of waking up very early in the morning. If you suspect that your problem is really one of a severely depressed mood, seek professional help.

It is understandable that tinnitus is more noticeable in the evening when all is quiet. The ambient sounds of the city reduce dramatically in the middle of the night when traffic diminishes to a trickle. At these times, tinnitus seems to become louder, and, like any other form of distraction, it can hinder sleep. However, it is puzzling that the ability to sleep is sometimes completely unaffected by tinnitus.

Before you blame tinnitus for any difficulty you may have in sleeping, consider other physical and psychological causes. Almost any illness can affect sleep, as can certain medications taken to treat illness. Caffeine in tea and coffee, and appetite supressants, may hinder sleep. If you have recently been bereaved you are unlikely to sleep as well. If you are inactive and take naps during the day you will naturally feel less sleepy at night. The amount of sleep a person needs to feel refreshed varies widely — the normal range is five to ten hours. The need for sleep often declines with age.

Physical dependence on sleeping tablets

Sleeping tablets become less effective over time if they are taken every night. After several months the need for them may be more apparent than real in the sense that a vicious cycle develops. As physical dependence grows, the action of stopping the tablets is almost sure to lead to a 'rebound' insomnia. As a result, a person begins to mistrust his ability to sleep and feels that it is essential to take the tablets. Any threat to withdraw them induces apprehension. The worry that sleep might not come then adds to the difficulty of getting to sleep.

If you want to stop taking sleeping tablets (or use them more sparingly), it is advisable to consult the doctor who prescribed them. I have found that there is sometimes confusion about why certain drugs have been prescribed, especially when a person is taking several different types of pill. Of course, not all drugs taken at night are sleeping tablets.

Withdrawal of sleeping tablets should be done gradually over several weeks. The reason for this is that withdrawal can lead to a temporary increase in insomnia, in anxiety feelings and in other side-effects. Balancing these negative effects, there should be some positive ones like feeling less drowsy during the day, performing your tasks with a clearer mind, and feeling less irritable.

Sleep without drugs

For a full description of psychological techniques, the reader is referred to books devoted to this subject. I will limit this section to an outline of general principles. Tinnitus brings with it its own special problems and I shall consider these too. If you set out to change your sleeping habits, record your success in a sleep diary; at a minimum this should list when you went to sleep and arose, and the frequency of night-time waking. In this way, you will be able to review your progress over a long time period.

General principles: getting off to sleep

- Go to bed sleepy. Do not try to get more sleep by going to bed early. Keep active during the day and do not take naps.
- Do not read, watch T.V., or eat in bed unless you are sure from past experience that these activities will help you to sleep.
- Do not think about getting to sleep or worry about the day's activities. Attempt instead to relax your muscles and think pleasant thoughts.

- If you are unable to fall asleep within 15 minutes, get up immediately and do something like reading in a different room. Return to bed only when sleepy.
- Set your alarm to get up at the same time each morning irrespective of how much sleep you received the night before.

Sleep cannot be willed, and so the main principle is *not* to try to get to sleep but to create the conditions in which sleep comes more easily. This means building up regular sleep habits, practising relaxation before going to bed, and using your bed for sleeping rather than a place to worry, read, or otherwise entertain yourself. So, if sleep fails to come after 15 minutes, it is suggested that you leave your bed and occupy yourself elsewhere, returning after 30 minutes. If once more sleep eludes you, the process is repeated, throughout the night if necessary.

Waking in the night

If your sleep is broken by frequent periods of wakefulness, it is not advisable to remain in bed worrying about not sleeping and thinking how tired you will be in the morning. Instead, go to a different room, make a drink if you feel like it, sit in a comfortable chair and do something that is not over-stimulating. Return to bed when you feel tired, and if sleep does not come within 15 minutes, repeat this cycle.

It may happen that a habit develops of waking at a certain time, say 2.30 a.m. This may be followed by a ritual visit to the toilet or making of a drink, by which time you are fully awake. Instead of following the urge to get up immediately, normal sleep can sometimes be achieved by remaining in bed for about 15 minutes while you engage in a relaxation exercise (see below). If this fails, the advice of getting up for 30 minutes should be followed.

Insomnia and tinnitus

It is common knowledge that loud noises stimulate us into wakefulness. We also know that it is possible to ignore loud noises if they are familiar and unimportant. A loud tinnitus may disturb sleep at first but later on a person adjusts to the presence of their noises and sleeps normally as before. Tinnitus may keep a person awake not because it is loud but because it is worrying and irritating.

One way of dealing with the intrusiveness of noises at night is to find a repetitive activity which at one and the same time distracts attention and partially masks your noise. A masker (see Chapter 10) worn in the evening before retiring can be of help in getting off to sleep. For a fortunate few, tinnitus is quieter after using it. An in-the-ear masker can also be worn at night without physical discomfort. Listening to the hiss of a radio tuned off-station (or, if you prefer, soothing music) is another possibility. A relaxation tape played at night in bed can serve the purpose of masking and distraction (althought, unfortunately, it might not be welcomed by your partner.) The problem of changing tapes can be solved with a continuous loop tape or auto-reverse recorder, or a long tape can be made and the recorder switched off by a time switch. Some radio/cassette alarm clocks have the facility of switching off at a pre-set time.

A method that distracts attention away from tinnitus, and is also relaxing, is the muscle tension/release method mentioned earlier. It will take some time to work through all the muscle groups if you take it slowly. The muscles should be tensed only slightly, just sufficient to be aware of the sensation. Then the muscle is relaxed and you concentrate on the warm tingling feeling you get as you do so. Work up from your toes to your head, following the instructions that you find in books on progressive muscular relaxation. If your mind wanders onto the tinnitus or worrying thoughts, bring it back to the tensing/relaxing task. I have been assured that this is better than counting sheep.

Final word

Some of the techniques I have described are little more than promising ideas; others have been evaluated and shown to be useful. As a general survey, the chapter may lack the detail you require. You might have difficulty applying general principles to your own particular circumstances. If so, you should read further to deepen your understanding (see Bibliography). Alternatively, a few sessions with a professional therapist might be sufficient to get you going on your own self-help programme. Tinnitus associations are also a valuable source of support through their local branch meetings (see Chapter 11).

If, after a fair attempt at coming to terms with tinnitus by yourself, you still feel that you are not progressing, do not hold back from seeking expert help. The techniques I have described in the last two chapters are *not* a panacea for all of life's stresses or for all the problems that tinnitus poses.

10
Modifying the environment

There are three main strategies for modifying the environment in order to ease the problem of tinnitus:

- *Attention-absorbing activities* — activities can be arranged that absorb your attention so that less time is spent listening to tinnitus.
- *Masking* — arranging for external sounds to cover up your head noises.
- *Changing the social environment* — asking your family and friends to react differently to you, or reacting differently to them so that tinnitus interferes less in your personal relationships.

Some of these strategies might not be available to you. For example, some head noises are too intense to be masked completely, and to wear a *tinnitus masker* (see later) your hearing needs to be good enough to hear the masking noise at a comfortable volume. Use of the other strategies may depend on the type of tinnitus you have, your living arrangements, and so on. It is likely that you will have to adapt these strategies to suit your personal circumstances.

Some environmental approaches combine several strategies. The provision of a hearing aid, if you have need of one, is a good example (see below).

Hearing and tinnitus

The auditory handicaps that often accompany tinnitus have been talked about in Chapter 2. It is possible that tinnitus itself will affect your ability to hear well, but without a proper audiological assessment it is difficult to decide whether tinnitus or hearing loss is primarily responsible for your hearing problems. A partial loss of hearing (for example, in one ear or at certain sound frequencies) is very common, and a hearing aid should be considered in such cases. If you are profoundly deaf, the environmental strategies available to you for influencing tinnitus are fewer in number. You will have to rely more on the methods described in Chapters 8 and 9.

Regarding the effect of environmental sound, there are two main types of tinnitus. One type, fortunately in the minority, gets louder after exposure to sound. Quietness is sought out because tinnitus is softer under these conditions. The other type is masked by external sounds and so quietness is avoided. However, the effects of external sounds greatly depend on their intensity, and an environment which is neither quiet nor loud may be preferred. Most people experience ringing in the ears after exposure to very loud noises and it is normal to avoid them.

Whether or not you continue to follow your normal work and social activities, or change them, depends on a variety of factors. I have known of clients who have moved house to get away from quietness — or to seek it out. For many, it is a question of balancing the enjoyment of, say, a theatre outing or party, against the loss of appreciation resulting from intrusive noise or difficulty in hearing. This balance may depend on your mood and the loudness of tinnitus at the time. If these are unpredictable, it can become difficult to plan ahead. It is important that your family and friends are aware that there may be moments when you feel like retiring completely from company, and that they accept your right to do this.

It hardly needs pointing out that a strategy of avoidance is two-edged. Without the stimulation and company of others, your thoughts are more likely to turn to tinnitus and its depressing effects. As a general rule, then, it is worth continuing as normal and tolerating, as far as possible, the undesirable effects of your auditory impairments.

Another phenomenon which may disturb you is an impression that everyday sounds are uncomfortably loud or reverberate in your head. This may develop into an aversion or even a phobia for certain types of sound (see later).

Hearing aids in tinnitus suppression

It is increasingly recognized that a hearing aid is worth trying as a first option in the management of tinnitus even though the degree of hearing loss would not normally warrant the fitting of an aid. Aids may be fitted for each ear when the hearing loss or the tinnitus is present bilaterally. As noted above, any difficulty you experience listening to others, especially in a group, is likely to be due to a mixture of hearing loss and intrusive tinnitus. However, tinnitus is the more obvious cause and it may get the blame unfairly. It has been found that, besides improving your hearing, an aid can decrease the troublesomeness of head noises. The aid assists with masking (see below) because there is some noise from the instrument itself and the sounds you want to hear above your tinnitus are enhanced as well. Hearing aids are generally less effective than maskers in covering up tinnitus, but the benefits of an aid may continue to be felt for a more extended period after the initial fitting.

Attention absorbing activities

The role of attention was explained in Chapters 5 and 6. One of the commonest ways of coping with tinnitus is to get involved in doing something that so grips your concentration that the noises are temporarily forgotten. If the activity makes a noise, so much the better. Banging away on an old-fashioned typewriter may do the trick, or any manual activity that absorbs your interest can be effective. I have found that it is mainly in the early stages of coming to terms with tinnitus that these strategies are employed. They provide temporary benefit only and, taken to extremes, they could exhaust you. As tolerance is acquired, the need for this strategy will lessen as you begin to notice that you have *not noticed* your tinnitus even at times of normal activity.

Masking

The principle of masking is that a louder sound covers up a quieter sound so that only the louder sound is heard. How does this apply to tinnitus? Noises in the head are generally quieter than external sounds and so they are often masked by the hubbub of traffic, office, and factory noise. It is only in quiet surroundings, perhaps at home in the evening, that they become noticeable. City dwellers who retire to their country retreat may begin to find tinnitus intruding into their peace and quiet.

The louder the tinnitus the less often environmental masking occurs. If your tinnitus varies in loudness you might get complete masking on some days and partial masking on others. The masking of one *external* sound by another is not exactly the same phenomenon as the masking of head noises. The former obeys simpler laws. The masking of one physical sound by another is an all-or-none phenomenon but head noises have the habit of breaking through a masking sound to become audible again. Perhaps this is because tinnitus is not a 'real' sound corresponding to a quantifiable physical force. When tinnitus breaks through a masking sound you will hear both noises at the same time. This 'partial masking' might still be preferable to none at all; at least the tinnitus is *relatively* less loud and therefore less noticeable.

The portable masking devices that are now commercially available produce a meaningless shushing sound, but similar benefits can be obtained from recorded voices or music that cover up your noise. Portable cassette recorders have a useful part to play in this respect. Enthusiasts of 'sound therapy' have recently been promoting the use of specially prepared tapes of classical music. These recordings, which retain more of the higher pitched sounds, are said to 'recharge and tone up' the brain. If you believe this you will also find that they release your unconscious fantasies and cure you of all manner of afflictions!

Finding the ideal form of environmental masking is a question of experiment. In the evening, meaningful masking sounds may be too stimulating and keep you awake. A radio tuned off station will produce a meaningless sound that may serve well enough. Of course, with a personal cassette recorder you have an endless choice of possible sounds to listen to — meaningful or meaningless. Some recorders have a graphic equalizer that allows you to emphasize some frequencies and cut out others. In this way you might achieve a more harmonious, effective or comforting sound. Alternatively, you can obtain a tinnitus masking device.

Acquiring a tinnitus masker

There are various explanations for the beneficial effects of wearing a tinnitus masker. It may work in different ways for different people and so, if you intend to acquire the device, it is important to understand what it can and cannot do for you. It is also important to have a masker fitted by a qualified dispenser, technician, or ear specialist. A hearing aid might give better results and, in any case, maskers are fitted with moulds specially made to insert into your external ear canal. These need to be properly vented so that external sounds are not prevented from entering the ear. You will require instruction in inserting the mould and adjusting the controls. Several visits may be needed to get everything right.

Tinnitus maskers became available just over ten years ago. The most popular device is worn behind the ear like a hearing aid and it delivers a hissing sound into the ear canal. The volume of the masking noise is adjustable and it is recommended that you use only the *minimum volume of sound* required for masking. Different models produce somewhat different noises (e.g. lower or higher pitch) and so it is worth experimenting to find the best one. You may have received the impression that a tinnitus masker is a form of treatment (that is, curative) but this is a misunderstanding. The device is simply a portable, unobtrusive source of sound. Put to service with the right expectations, a masker can help you to learn to live with tinnitus. As I mentioned earlier, the device is not suitable for someone whose hearing is very poor or in cases where tinnitus is not maskable. Often it is simply a matter of giving the device a fair trial. It is normally worn in the ear in which the tinnitus is heard or appears loudest. However, it will also work effectively if the noises are heard in the centre of the head or if it is worn in a 'good' ear to mask tinnitus heard in the other. Maskers are sometimes supplied for both ears, especially when the tinnitus is heard in the centre of the ear or, naturally, in both ears.

It is not necessary to use a masker indefinitely; it is intended more as a way of coping with noises in the early stages of adjustment. After a while, frequency of use typically falls off. However, this depends on how the masker works for you and what pattern of use suits you.

Your initial reaction to wearing a masker might be quite negative but you should not reject it out of hand. In the first place, a brief trial in the clinic where you try it out is unlike your home environment. Secondly, you should have the opportunity for a prolonged period of use — at least an hour a day for, say, four weeks. Purchase of a device should be delayed until you are sure you want it.

It is recommended that the volume control be set so that the masking sound just covers your noise. If this is uncomfortably loud, the volume can be set at a lower level for partial masking only. A regular pattern of use is advisable. In other words, do not simply use it when tinnitus is most bothersome. Under these conditions the masker might not make a substantial difference to your mood, in which case you are unlikely to develop confidence in it. Furthermore there *are* good reasons for suggesting regular use (see below).

Explanations given for masker benefit

1. *Habituation of attention.* This process was described in Chapters 5 and 6. It is easier to ignore (switch attention away from) noises that are constant and meaningless. So, if instead of hearing your tinnitus you hear a constant hiss, it will be easier to place your attention elsewhere. Another way of putting this is to say that the masking noise is more acceptable. This is often the case when your noise has an unpleasant high pitched tone. Masking sounds have even be described by some tinnitus experts as having a soothing and mildly tranquillizing effect.

2. *Personal control.* Research has sown that unpleasant noises are more tolerable when you have some control over them — even if this is a *possibility* for control which is never exercised. Thus, one explanation for why the masking sound is more tolerable is that you have complete control over its volume and timing. It allows you to take a rest from your own noises and hear something different. It gives you the feeling that at least *something* can be done when the noise is extremely annoying.

3. *Residual inhibition.* In a small proportion of users, the effects of masking persist after the device has been switched off. Complete disappearance of tinnitus is rare (7 per cent of users in one study) although a partial quieting of the noise is more common. Unfortunately, the residual effects are not long-lasting and will probably be counted in minutes or hours. The effect is sometimes sufficiently powerful to influence the pattern of masker use. When inhibition is present, use of the masker can be limited to an hour or so in early morning and late evening. It is said that residual inhibition is more likely to occur after certain types of masking noise than others. It is therefore necessary to experiment with masking sounds or tones of different pitches to discover whether

this is so. In order to produce residual inhibition the masking noise is turned up to a raised volume (that is, above the minimal masking level) for a short period of time. Residual inhibition should be regarded as an extra bonus from the masker, not its main function. Disappearance of the tinnitus for a few minutes does not mean that the masker has 'cured' your noises.

Types of wearable device

Behind-the-ear. Looks like and is worn like a hearing aid (see description above). Different models have somewhat different sound characteristics and power.

In-the-ear (ear canal) masker. This fits straight onto an ear mould or standard base so there is no behind the ear device. It can be fitted easily and quickly and is comfortable even when the wearer is lying in bed.

Combination instrument (or tinnitus instrument). A combined hearing aid and masker. There are several types including an in-the-ear model. They require more skill in fitting than a simple masker and in some models the controls are difficult to operate. If the hearing aid and masking functions are not required at the same time a separate aid and masker may be more practical. The procedure for adjusting the controls is always to set the volume control on the hearing aid first and then to add in the masking sound. In this way, masking can be achieved at a lower volume.

Programmable masker. This is a body-worn device with head phones which can be programmed to deliver a sound chosen as the most satisfactory on the basis of previous tests. The point of this is that a masking sound can be selected which is quieter, more acceptable, or produces more residual inhibition.

What is the evidence that maskers are helpful?

Unfortunately, a straightforward answer to this question cannot be given because some people reject the idea of a masker out of hand or, even when open to it, find the masking noise as annoying as their own tinnitus. When masking devices were first distributed by post in Britain on a casual basis less than one in ten users were helped.

Since then, masking devices have been fitted with greater care and with clear indications of what to expect from the instrument. Counselling and follow-up appointments are usually offered. Belief in the value of masking varies from clinic to clinic, but a recommendation for trial use may be made in up to 50 per cent of cases. About 20 per cent of people recommended a masker refuse to try it and another 20 per cent discontinue after a trial period (these figures depend on whether the masker is supplied free or has to be purchased). The proportion who eventually obtain some benefit is usually less than a quarter of those offered one. To some extent these figures might reflect the fact that the user's expectations of the device are wrong or over-optimistic.

In a recent large-scale British study, 40-60 per cent of eventual users said that their tinnitus was inaudible when the masker was worn. The comparable figure for those who were prescribed a hearing aid was 20 per cent.

Research has been conducted to compare the benefits of masker fitting with alternative forms of help. In one trial, as much help was obtained from an impressive looking device that supposedly delivered a weak electric current to the ear. In another, the benefits of counselling alone were greater in some respects than the provision of a masker. For these reasons, one cannot be sure that all the help coming from masker use is actually coming from the masker.

It is not sensible to draw too sweeping a conclusion from these findings. A person who attends a tinnitus clinic probably obtains reassurance from a variety of sources, even from the knowledge that someone is trying to be helpful. As long as tinnitus maskers are helping a minority, they are worth providing for those who can obtain benefit. It is also fair to say that first reactions to the masker are not necessarily a good guide to what can be achieved after a reasonable trial. Unfortunately, research has not yet given us many clues as to who is likely to benefit and who is not.

The safety of maskers. While there is no evidence of maskers causing a deterioration of hearing through excessive exposure to sound, this is no reason for complacency. The limit of safety for long-term exposure to environmental sound is around 85-90 decibels, but the maximum output of some maskers exceeds that level. Of course, maskers are not normally worn on maximum volume but the initial level that is set sometimes proves ineffective, so the user ends up 'chasing his tinnitus' with higher masking levels. Rather than risk using the masker on maximum output, it might be preferable to settle for partial masking or use it when the tinnitus is at a moderate (and maskable) intensity.

The same caution applies to using a portable cassette recorder (Walkman). In a recent study, 20 per cent of users (who were mostly normally-hearing school children) reported symptoms of tinnitus or dullness of hearing after using the recorder. If these effects are experienced, the authors advise reducing the volume or duration of listening.

The masker as a desensitization device. There is some evidence to show that people who are bothered by tinnitus are more intolerant of loud noises in general. As the intensity of an external sound is increased, a person who has tinnitus will more quickly reach the point of uncomfortable loudness. There are several ways of explaining this. It could be that noise intolerance is a life-long characteristic in some individuals who would, for this reason, be more liable to annoyance from tinnitus.

Another possibility is that a person who has an ear disorder becomes more sensitive to sounds and experiences the phenomenon of *loudness recruitment* mentioned earlier. When hearing loss is present, the spectrum of quiet to loud sounds is compressed into a smaller range of physical sound pressures, especially at levels that are close to the threshold of hearing. This means that even a small change in air pressure can produce a sudden and unpleasant increase in loudness. This is something that you may have noticed if you developed a hearing loss in adult life.

One more explanation is that a person who is bothered by tinnitus has been traumatized by loud sounds in the past and retains a fear of noise. This can happen to a child exposed at an early age to bursting balloons or fireworks. In adulthood the cause is more likely to be wartime bombing. When the fear is extreme, the term phonophobia applies. (There are also aversions to *quiet* sounds such as the crackle of newspaper, the sound of ironing, chalk on a blackboard, clicking of false teeth, which probably have a different origin).

In cases of loudness sensitivity the masker can be valuable as a tool for desensitization (this was pointed out to me by J. Hazell). One method of desensitization involves exposing yourself to things you fear. In the case of noises, the general principle is gradual exposure to louder and louder sounds for longer and longer periods. It is important, however, to start with a very low volume and short exposure (30-60 minutes) and not to proceed to a higher level or longer durations until the preceding setting is tolerated with comfort. Although the idea is speculative, it is possible that some of the benefits of masker use result from a process of desensitization.

Changing your social environment

Your tinnitus not only affects you, it also affects indirectly the people around you. As I have mentioned before, tinnitus does not readily elicit sympathy, or at least not for long. Others may have to be reminded to make allowances. You should not feel that the invisibility of head noises diminishes your right to be affected by them. One man told me that the chief benefit he obtained from a masker was its audibility to other people. His family quickly got the message when the noises were troublesome. It is perhaps easy to discount your noises and begin to feel that you are a burden. However, other people do *not* know what it is like to hear your noises and who is to say how they would cope in your shoes. It is important to give the people who are close to you an opportunity to read up on the subject. It is also instructive to play them a hissing sound (say from a radio) which is matched to the loudness of your own noises.

However, I am more concerned in this section with the situation that can arise if tinnitus leads to a deterioration in your personal relationships. A dilemma arises from the fact that a sympathetic gesture can remind you of your tinnitus when your general aim is to regard the noises as *less* significant. The less often others remind you of your noises, the less often you are likely to remind *yourself* of them and hence notice them. If you have got into the habit of thinking of yourself as a 'tinnitus sufferer' and others reinforce this idea, you have got yourself into a thinking trap. Conversation turns far too readily to this topic.

There is no simple solution to this dilemma: you may have to take the bull by the horns and just act differently. To ease your way into a new way of thinking you can opt initially to act as though you were your normal self, a 'non-sufferer', for perhaps a half day or evening. It helps to do something out of the ordinary (for you) at this time. In any event, all mention of tinnitus should be forbidden and this should be agreed in advance. I hope you will be pleasantly surprised by the result.

As I have declared time and again in this book, it is possible to lead a normal life in spite of tinnitus. Your attempts to deal with the problem should be indirect and, as it were, 'off the cushion', but be confident that you will get there in the end.

11
A glance into the future

When we look into the future it is usually with an optimistic eye. The hoped-for cure for tinnitus is surely not far away. Some of my clients express surprise that medical research has not yet come up with the final answer. I respond by saying that tinnitus is not the symptom of any single disorder; therefore, many cures will be needed. In fact some causes of tinnitus (which apply in only a minority of cases) are already treatable. Sadly, in some cases, treating the disorder which causes tinnitus still leaves the symptom as it was — the damage has already been done. Moreover, our understanding of the *physiological mechanisms* in ear and brain that produce tinnitus is still speculative. Until they are understood, the elimination of all tinnitus is a distant prospect.

The most hopeful sign is that medical and research interest is growing. There have been three international conferences on tinnitus since 1979, spaced at four-yearly intervals. More are planned. The contributors have looked at the subject from all possible angles. A research newsletter has grown out of these contacts and it is being distributed internationally. If significant advances are made anywhere in the world, you can be assured that the news will spread rapidly.

In the meantime, our developing knowledge of the causes of tinnitus should be used in efforts to lower the incidence of new cases. A common cause is excessive exposure to loud sound. The harmful effect on hearing is well recognized, and legislation has been introduced in many countries to limit preventable damage. The link with tinnitus has taken second place but the number of claims in the courts against employers on account of noise-induced tinnitus is now growing. These claims have created a legal tangle because tinnitus is a subjective phenomenon and, unlike hearing loss, its effects are largely unquantifiable.

When one reflects on the noises generated in everyday life, including excessive volumes of amplified music, it has to be concluded that noise pollution is not taken very seriously. Ear protectors are not always worn when they are provided in compliance with regulations. It should be noted that the effects of excessive noise are cumulative. Until the public is made more aware of harmful levels of exposure to noise, tinnitus is likely to be an increasing problem in the future. Of course, it hardly needs saying that if noise exposure has been a significant factor in your case, you should protect yourself with ear muffs or ear plugs against further damage from loud sounds such as chain-saws, outboard motors, and industrial machines.

Are there, then, any hopeful signs in the medical field? I can do no better than quote from the remarks of Ellis Douek who gave the final summing up at the last international conference (1987) at Munster, West Germany. He announced his conclusions with some trepidation. Surgery, he said, has 'a limited place'. Drug therapy 'remains in the same situation in which it has been for a while.' He foresaw 'continual development' in the application of masking, and interesting prospects for electrical stimulation. In the light of this sober appraisal, it was not surprising to hear him concluding that 'psychological efforts, broadly speaking, remain the basis of our management of these patients and there is no doubt that we will have to continue to discuss the best approach.' He did not mean by this, I am sure, that patients should be given compassionless exhortations to 'learn to live with it.' Efforts have to be made on all fronts, and as long as curative treatments remain unavailable, we should try to understand the basis of tinnitus distress and find out what can be done to alleviate it.

The psychological approach has already been discussed at length in this book so I will not attempt to look any further into the future. Some readers might consider the approach experimental enough as it is. A healthy sign, however, is that determined efforts are being made to evaluate the psychological methods I have described.

Developments in masking

Masking technology remains in the forefront of medical attention. However, the first flush of enthusiasm has died away to leave a more realistic appraisal of the valuable, but not necessarily central, role of tinnitus masking. In one New York clinic, purchase of masking devices has declined in the last few years, but fewer people are returning them. This seems to indicate a better appreciation of the uses and limitations of maskers. Increased efforts are now being made to tailor the masking noise to individual needs. The purpose is to find a masker that produces maximum coverage of the tinnitus at minimum volume and with minimum interference with hearing. Other considerations are the acceptability of the noise and the maximization of residual inhibition effects. It is fair to say that these are refinements to an existing technology and not a radical change of direction.

Electrical stimulation

Electrical stimulation via skin electrodes has proved effective in suppressing pain sensations and applications to tinnitus are now being explored. The first attempts to stimulate the ear electrically date back to 1801 shortly after Volta developed his battery. In spite of its long history, there is a great deal to find out about the safety and effectiveness of electrical stimulation.

Electrode placement is important. The area around the ear is one popular site but stimulation to the middle ear, nearer to the cochlea, is probably more effective. Medical researchers are investigating the type of current that produces greatest suppression and they are also looking carefully at side-effects such as tissue damage, pain, dizziness, and unwanted auditory sensations. Studies of the effects of short-term stimulation (using very weak currents of course) have produced some encouraging results, but the practicability of long-term use remains questionable.

If a safe and effective technique could be found it would be of especial value to the profoundly deaf who cannot benefit from masking. In fact, tinnitus suppression has been noticed in a number of profoundly deaf individuals who have been given a cochlear implant. An implant is a device that electrically stimulates the inner ear producing auditory sensations that correspond in part with sounds in the real world. Cochlear implants are not normally offered to a person who has some useful hearing as this would be sacrificed in the implant operation. The potential of cochlear implantation for tinnitus suppression is still very uncertain.

The role of voluntary organizations

It is fitting to end this book, and this chapter, by looking at the present and future role of voluntary organizations. Tinnitus associations are well established in some countries and are springing up in others. This development echoes a general trend for medical consumers to lobby for better services and to promote support groups for individuals with particular disorders.

Voluntary organizations come into existence when it is obvious that there are commonly felt unmet needs. Local interest groups are usually established following public meetings which provoke awareness of those needs and draw attention to possible solutions. The British Tinnitus Association (BTA) was formed after a radio broadcast by Jack Ashley, a well-known Member of Parliament, in which he described his own deafness and tinnitus. The BTA now consists of over 100 local groups dotted around the country linked by a central office and newsletter. The American Tinnitus Association (ATA) with over 150 groups is said to have a mailing list of 140,000 names and to have 20,000 subscribers. One of the main functions of national organizations is to collect and disseminate information.

Local tinnitus groups vary in size and energy. Usually there is a member who arranges a place to meet, a programme of guest speakers, and a communication link such as a newsletter. Apart from the facilitator, the groups do not normally have a leader. However, within the group are members who have adapted to their tinnitus and have a great deal of useful advice and experience to pass on to new members. Some are acknowledged as lay counsellors who are willing to listen to distressed members over the telephone or even visit them at home. A high proportion of the tinnitus population are elderly people living alone, possessing limited financial resources. Group support is valuable in these circumstances. This is not to imply that all tinnitus group members are elderly. Groups catering for a much younger age band have also been set up in some places.

Self-help groups do not appeal to everyone but they do have a considerable amount to offer. Their members may have got little satisfaction from professionals, or the advice they received may not have been to their liking. Many of them had been told that there was no cure or way of alleviating their symptoms but this was not followed up by adequate counselling. A complete assessment and treatment of tinnitus requires contributions from many disciplines. Apart from the medical ear specialist and audiologist, the services of a nutritionist, psychologist, chiropractor, allergist, or psychiatrist could be relevant in particular cases. However, the professionals don't always agree among themselves. For this reason, or through lack of knowledge, one specialist might not refer a client to another specialist.

For some individuals, the idea of taking control of their own lives is more appealing than seeking professional help. Indeed, the tinnitus group member who experiences noises and has lived through a process of adaptation has a source of informal knowledge on which to draw and share. In many ways, the indigenous expert is more knowledgeable and more persuasive than the professional. Newly affected sufferers can draw strength from a group member who has witnessed at first hand the reality of the growth of tolerance. Moreover, in contrast to the frequent lack of interest shown by family and friends, fellow club members are willing to share experiences, discuss them, and offer reassurance about fears that would be difficult to express in less secure surroundings. Surprise is often expressed at the discovery that not everyone is affected in the same way by noises. This underlines the realization that the origins and remedy for distress lie within the individual.

New members also get tips on how to contend with the effects of tinnitus, on the use of maskers and hearing aids, and on other specific points. They may be prompted into seeking specialist opinions by more experienced members who recognize the need for this. In short, a well-running tinnitus group is a source of good counsel and hope.

Of course, not all groups are so constructive. Some do not manage to provide a climate of trust and openness. There may be too many members who want to unburden their distress and too few indigenous experts to inculcate a feeling of optimism. In some instances, members who have learned to cope are disparaging of others who are still struggling. Moreover, groups are unlikely to be beneficial to members if discussion focuses exclusively on remedies and the possibility of cure. Tinnitus has so many different causes that what is effective for one member may be totally ineffective for another. Furthermore, some diets and drugs could be harmful to individuals with certain medical disorders,

The occasional drawbacks of mutual help groups are greatly outweighed by their advantages. It is also worth entertaining two other potential arrangements which fall between individual professional advice and non-directed mutual help. The first is the directed group led by someone who has expertise in a particular area. The group may be designed to have a limited life, but long enough to impart certain skills such as cognitive techniques or relaxation. Alternatively, the group might be of the open-ended, drop-in type, but led by a facilitator skilled in fostering a supportive and empathetic group response when upsetting experiences are discussed.

Directed groups have several advantages. For example, individuals who are most likely to profit by the group can be selected initially. When the group begins to operate, the leader will be on the alert for participants who might be better served by individual therapy or by specialized audiological rehabilitation. If the leader has a broad knowledge of tinnitus and its management, he or she will be able to answer questions about worrying matters or the appropriateness of this or that treatment.

The directed groups I have been discussing could be located either in a hospital clinic/audiology centre or arranged by a tinnitus association in collaboration with a group leader it chooses to employ. An entirely different development for the future is for lay counsellors to enhance their counselling skills through additional training. Some form of support or training for lay counsellors is, in any case, advisable in order to safeguard against exploitation, burnout, or failure to detect problems that could be alleviated in other ways. Counselling, whether provided by trained or untrained individuals, is a responsible and demanding activity. Altruism and fellow-feeling are praiseworthy and often in scarce supply. However, lay counsellors could find themselves overwhelmed if they do not place limits on their availability. It would be helpful, in any additional training, for lay counsellors to receive guidance on picking out the person who really does need specialized therapy. This would avoid the situation of a few very needy individuals draining away the scarce energies of the counsellor. Thus, it is important that lay counsellors establish links with a network of local services and feel that they can consult freely with professionals.

Tinnitus is such a common disorder that the ear specialist or related professional can hope to do little more than offer a service when self-help, mutual help, or routine medical advice have proved inadequate. I hope this book goes some way towards making it easier for you to tap into your own resources, to know when to seek advice, and to make use of it when you get it.

Bibliography

General Reading

CIBA Foundation Symposium 85. (Evered, D. & Lawrenson, G., Eds), *Tinnitus*, Pitman: London, 1981.

Clark, J. G. & Yanick, P., (Eds), *Tinnitus and its management*, C.C. Thomas: Springfield, Ill., 1984.

Hallam, R. S., Rachman, S. & Hinchcliffe, R., 'Psychological aspects of tinnitus' *Contributions to medical psychology*, Vol 3, Pergamon Press: Oxford, 1984.

Hazell, J. W. P., (Ed), *Tinnitus*, Churchill Livingstone: Edinburgh, 1987.

McFadden, D., *Tinnitus: Facts, theories, & treatments*, Working Group 89, National Research Council, National Academy Press: Washington, D. C., 1982.

Proceedings of 1st International Tinnitus Seminar, New York, June 1979, *Journal of Laryngology and Otology*, Supplement No.4, 1981.

Proceedings of 2nd International Tinnitus Seminar, New York, June 1983, *Journal of Laryngology and Otology*, Supplement, 1985.

Proceedings of 3rd International Tinnitus Seminar, Munster, 1987, Feldmann, H., (Ed), Harsch Verlag: Karlsruhe, 1987.

Slater, R., & Terry, M. *Tinnitus: A guide for sufferers and professionals*, Croom Helm: London, 1987.

Relaxation/suggestion

Benson, A. *The relaxation response*, Collins, Fontana paperbacks: Glasgow, 1977.

Horn, S., *Relaxation: Modern techniques for stress management*, Thorsons: Wellingborough, 1986.

Young, P., *Personal change through self-hypnosis*, Angus and Robertson: London, 1986.

Cognitive techniques

Blackburn, I., *Coping with depression*, Chambers: Edinburgh, 1987.

Burns, D. D., *Feeling Good*, New American Library: New York, 1980.

Glossary

This glossary contains terms that you are likely to encounter in your further reading. Most of them have not appeared in this book because it has not been my intention to provide an account of the medical or audiological aspects of tinnitus.

Acoustic emissions
Sounds emitted by the cochlea which can be detected with a very sensitive microphone placed in the ear canal. These are normal and not the basis of tinnitus.

Audiogram
This is a graph of your threshold of hearing (qv) at different sound frequencies. It is usually shown as hearing loss in dB units. O dB represents the normal threshold of hearing.

Auricle
The visible part of the ear.

Basilar membrane
A membrane inside the cochlea (qv) that is set into vibration by the action of sound waves on the eardrum and ossicles (qv). Movement of the membrane leads to the production of neural impulses in the auditory nerve.

Binaural
Pertaining to both ears.

Cochlea
A spiral fluid-filled tube divided into two chambers situated in the inner ear. It contains the sensory organ of hearing which consists of special nerve-endings of the cochlear nerve, called hair

cells, capable of detecting the frequency and amplitude of vibrations in the surrounding fluid.

Cochlear implant
A surgically implanted device for people who once had good hearing but have since become totally deaf. It incorporates a microphone and transforms sound into electrical impulses which are led into the ear to stimulate it directly. This does not produce 'normal hearing' but the auditory sensations are nonetheless of value in interpreting speech and other sounds.

Combination instrument (tinnitus instrument)
A combined hearing aid and tinnitus masker.

Conductive hearing loss
Deafness resulting from damage or disease of the middle ear (qv).

Decibel (dB)
A measurement unit for sound pressure. It is a logarithmic measure of the ratio of one pressure against a reference power. A change of 10 dB is usually perceived as a doubling of loudness.

Ear canal (internal auditory meatus)
The external canal or 'ear-hole' leading to the eardrum.

Eardrum (tympanic membrane)
The membrane situated at the end of the ear canal which vibrates with changes in sound pressure.

Earmould
A piece of resin individually made to fit the ear canal; it carries sound from the hearing aid or masker towards the eardrum.

Electrical suppression
The suppression of tinnitus by stimulating the ear with an electric current, delivered either externally or internally.

Eustachian tube
A tube connecting the air-filled middle ear to the back of the nose, thereby serving to equalize the pressure on each side of the eardrum. It opens up during chewing, swallowing or yawning movements.

Evoked acoustic emission (cochlear echo)
An acoustic emission (qv) responding to a tone played into the ear.

Glue ear
A common condition of childhood, but found in adults too, resulting from closure of the eustachian tube and accumulation of fluid in the middle ear. Hearing is affected, usually only temporarily. It may be treated surgically with grommets (qv).

Grommet
A small drainage tube surgically placed in the eardrum to remove fluid trapped in the middle ear.

Hair cells
Sensitive cells of the inner ear which transform sound vibrations into electrical (neural) impulses.

Hearing level (dB HL)
The threshold of hearing for a pure tone at a specified frequency relative to the normal hearing standard.

Hertz (Hz)
A unit of frequency equivalent to cycles per second.

Hyperacusis
An abnormal degree of discomfort or aversion to sounds that would not be regarded as loud by average standards.

Inner ear (labyrinth)
A fluid-filled sac comprising the organ of hearing (cochlea) and the organ of balance (the vestibule with its three semicircular canals).

Masking
The capacity of one sound to mask perception of another (quieter) sound. The greater the intensity of a sound the greater its masking effect.

Ménières disease
A condition of the inner ear giving rise to recurrent episodes of vertigo, usually associated with tinnitus, nausea or vomiting, and fluctuating hearing loss in one or both ears.

Middle ear
An air-filled chamber in which sound is conducted from the eardrum across the ossicles (qv) to the inner ear.

Monaural
Pertaining to one ear.

Neuroma (acoustic neuroma)
A small slow-growing tumour on the 8th cranial nerve which is rarely malignant but may have to be removed if it is compressing the nerve.

Noise-induced tinnitus
Tinnitus that is caused by overexposure to environmental sounds. Sudden impulse sounds such as gunshots and explosions are especially liable to cause damage.

Objective (vibratory) tinnitus
A relatively uncommon form of tinnitus which, if loud, can be heard by another person. If quiet, it can be detected by a sensitive microphone. It is normally heard as a click, pulse or hum. The cause is usually reflex muscular contractions or turbulence in blood vessels.

Organ of Corti
A part of the inner ear situated between the two coiled chambers of the cochlea, largely made up of hair cells (qv).

Ossicles (ossicular chain)
Three small bones in the middle ear (the hammer or malleus, anvil or incus, and stirrup or stapes) which transmit vibrations from the ear drum to a membrane of the cochlea.

Otitis externa
Inflammation of the ear canal causing itching; sometimes due to an underlying skin condition.

Otitis media
A term covering a variety of middle ear infections that cause the lining of the middle ear to become inflamed and secrete fluid.

Otosclerosis
A disease, in part hereditary, affecting the bones of the middle ear. The transmission of sound is affected producing a conductive hearing loss.

Ototoxic substance
A chemical substance (e.g. food or drug) having the effect of damaging the organ of hearing.

Oval window
A small oval membrane which is the point of contact between the ossicular chain and the inner ear.

Palatal myoclonus
Rythmic contraction of the muscles situated in the soft palate which may result in a clicking tinnitus.

Pitch
The perceptual quality of sounds of different frequency.

Presbyacusis
A term for the general loss of hearig that occurs with the ageing process, usually most pronounced in the higher frequencies.

Pulsatile tinnitus
Tinnitus taking the form of a regular pulsing sound. The pulse sometimes corresponds to the pulsing of blood in a vessel near the ear.

Recruitment (loudness recruitment)
Refers to the phenomenon in which even small increases in sound pressure cause disproportionate perception of loudness.

Residual inhibition
Refers to a lessening or cessation of tinnitus following delivery of an above-threshold external sound.

Semi-circular canals
The part of the inner ear concerned with balance and the ability to stand upright.

Sensation level (SL)
The intensity of a sound in relation to your own hearing threshold. Thus the same sound will have different sensation levels for people with different degrees of hearing loss.

Sensorineural hearing loss (nerve deafness)
Hearing loss caused by damage or disease of the sensory or neural elements of the auditory system (i.e. the cochlea and its neural connections.)

Sensorineural tinnitus
Tinnitus caused by disorder of the inner ear and its neural connections.

Speech audiogram
A graph indicating the ability to hear pre-recorded lists of words presented to the person through headphones at different intensities.

Stapedectomy
An operation for otosclerosis in which one of the middle ear bones (ossicles) is replaced by a tiny plastic piston.

Syringing
A method of removing excess wax by syringing water into the ear canal.

Threshold of hearing
The lowest intensity at which a pure tone can be detected (normally presented in a sound-insulated room.)

Tinnitus masker
An electronic device that feeds sound into the ear, and designed to cover up tinnitus noises.

Tympanic membrane
See eardrum.

Vertigo
A form of dizziness in which there is a sensation of the world spinning, or yourself spinning in relation to the world.

Useful addresses

List of national tinnitus associations and contact addresses:

Australia
Australian Tinnitus Association Ltd.,
288 Unwins Bridge Road
Sydenham
New South Wales 2044

Canada
Mrs E. Eayrs, Co-ordinator
The Tinnitus Association of Canada
23 Ellis Park Road
Toronto
Ontario M6S 2V4

Victoria Tinnitus Association
c/o Helen Caine
Western Institute for the Deaf
835 Humboldt Street, Room 302
Victoria, BC
V8V 2Z6

Germany
Deutsche Tinnitus-Liga C.V.
Lohsiepenstrasse 18
D-5600 Wuppertal 21
West Germany

New Zealand
Mrs J. Saunders B.A., M.A.,
New Zealand Tinnitus Association
31 William Souter Street
Forrest Hill
Auckland

Sweden
Tinnitusföreningen i Göteborg
Hörselrehabilileringen
Första Länggatan 30
413 27 Göteborg, Sweden

Tinnitussekfionen
Per. Olof Asp estrand
Norrley Tuärgata 11-13
502 64 Boras, Sweden

United Kingdom
British Tinnitus Association
105 Gower Street
London WC1E 6AH

USA
American Tinnitus Association
PO Box 5
Portland
Oregon 97207

Index